Step by Step

Injection Techniques in Orthopaedics

System requirement:

- **Windows XP or above**
- **Power DVD player (Software)**
- **Windows media player 10.0 version or above (Software)**

Accompanying CD ROM is playable only in Computer and not in CD player.

Step by Step

Injection Techniques in Orthopaedics

John Ebnezar

MMBS, D'Ortho, DNB (Ortho), MNAMS (Ortho), DAc, DMT

Consulting Orthopaedic and Spine Surgeon and Holistic Orthopaedic Expert

Formerly

Assistant Professor of Orthopaedics
Devaraj Urs Medical College
Kolar, Karnataka

Senior Specialist in Orthopaedics
Department of Orthopaeidics
Victoria Hospital
Bangalore Medical College

Presently

Chairman
The Physical Handicapped and
Paraplegic Charitable Trust of Karnataka ®

President
The Karnataka Orthopaedic Academy ®

Director
Bangalore Holistic Orthopaedic Centre, Bangalore

Medical Director
Parimala Hospital and Research Centre, Bangalore

Chairman
Ebnezar Institute of Orthopaedics, Bangalore

Jaypee Brothers

Wolters Kluwer Health | Lippincott Williams & Wilkins

First published in India in 2007 by
Jaypee Brothers Medical Publishers (P) Ltd, New Delhi, India.
EMCA House, 23/23B Ansari Road, Daryaganj, New Delhi 110 002, India
Phones: +91-11-23272143, +91-11-23272703, +91-11-23282021
Fax: +91-11-23276490, +91-11-23245683
e-mail: jaypee@jaypeebrothers.com
Visit our website: www.jaypeebrothers.com

First published in USA by The Lippincott Williams & Wilkins, 530 Walnut Street, Philadelphia, PA 19106, USA. Exclusively worldwide distributor except South East Asia (India, Nepal, Sri Lanka, Bhutan, Pakistan, Bangladesh).

ISBN 978-0-7817-9126-7

to

My mother (Late) Sampath Kumari
who taught me that life is more than self and
there is more joy in giving and
sharing than taking

My wife Dr Parimala, my lovely children
Rakesh and Priyanka
who are an epitome of love, sacrifice,
encouragement and inspiration

All my teachers
who made me what I am today
&
All my students past and present

Preface

Injection techniques in orthopaedics occupy a special place in the treatment armamentarium of orthopaedics. Injection techniques are an art and like all skills needs to be learnt methodically and diligently. But unfortunately, we as orthopaedic surgeons are never trained to give injections properly and no separate teaching programme is held for this unlike the training programme for surgeries, plaster techniques, traction, etc.

Most of the injection methods are learnt haphazardly just by observing some seniors and other staff. So, there is every chance of one picking up the improper and wrong techniques. Moreover, injection techniques are useful in a variety of orthopaedics disorders and not only a select few conditions like OA knee, low backache, calcaneal spurs and plantar fascitis, tennis elbow, etc.

So, to bridge these lacunae, I have put all my knowledge and experience of injection techniques in the form of a book. Hope the postgraduate students, junior orthopaedic surgeons and even senior surgeons will find this book useful and informative.

The book has been divided into four sections and deals with injection techniques in various conditions in each section. Your feedback is vital in improving upon the deficiencies in content and techniques in the forthcoming editions.

John Ebnezar

Acknowledgements

This book is the result of a team work involving the staff of my hospital. I would like to thank Dr Yogita, my junior assistant, Ravi, our senior OT staff, Kala, and Yogesh without whose help and cooperation it would have been virtually impossible for me to bring out this book.

I thank my wife Dr Parimala, my children Rakesh and Priyanka for their support and encouragement. I also thank Shri Jitendar P Vij and the entire team of M/s Jaypee Brothers Medical Publishers (P) Ltd., New Delhi for their full-fledged support and cooperation. They have done an excellent job and their effort is there for all to see.

I thank all my patients and also God for his kindness and grace which has kept me alive and kicking and has made me what I am today.

Contents

Section 1

Introduction to Injection Techniques

INTRODUCTION

Injections have always fascinated me. I have seen many patients yearning for that one wonder shot into the arm or buttocks, which can revert a patient from the gloom and despair of ill health to the comfort of normal health. I have always wondered how this unpleasant painful prick can restore normalcy in a jiffy. It took me some years of experience to realize that it mainly acted as a morale booster kindling a feeling of well-being in the patient that more often than not that did the trick and not its actual therapeutic effects.

However, there is a small group that is averse to the painful discomfiture an injection provides. Children in particular jump out of their skins at the very mention of the word injection. While the child cries its lungs out on being pricked, the parents seen to believe that louder the cry of their child faster will the disease flee from their beloved! A doctor with an injection in his hand appear as a villain to the child while he appears as a Messiah to the parents. This is the magic of injection in the field of medicine.

ROLE OF INJECTION IN ORTHOPAEDICS

The routine intramuscular and intravenous injection do find a place in orthopaedics in treating the fractures, dislocations, injections, arthritis, tumours, etc. Through these routes an orthopaedician seeks to administer painkillers, anaesthetics, intravenous fluids, blood, antibiotics, etc. to help him combat the orthopaedic disorders. However in orthopaedics apart from these routine techniques there are a few specialized injection techniques quite peculiar and specific to orthopaedic-related problems. Unlike the conventional injections, injections in orthopaedics can play a dual interesting role of diagnosis and treatment. This is what makes the injection in orthopaedics very special and interesting. It is a specialized skill that needs to be developed with lots of diligence and practice in the backdrop of sound bony anatomy and landmarks. Needless to say it is not everybody's cup of tea!

THE PURPOSE OF INJECTIONS IN ORTHOPAEDICS

The Diagnostic Role

Aspiration of the synovial fluid and diagnostic injections are the diagnostic techniques commonly employed in orthopaedics to make a diagnosis in specific cases.

a. *Diagnostic aspiration of the synovial fluid:* Examination of the aspirated synovial fluid helps confirm the diagnosis of different types of arthritis and also helps identify whether the disease is inflammatory or non-inflammatory.
b. *Diagnostic injection techniques:* This helps to:
   - Identify the source of pain
   - Indicate the exact area of the problem
   - Sort out the confusion regarding the diagnosis
   - Confirm the diagnosis
   - Provides a helpful guide to the future course of therapeutic action.

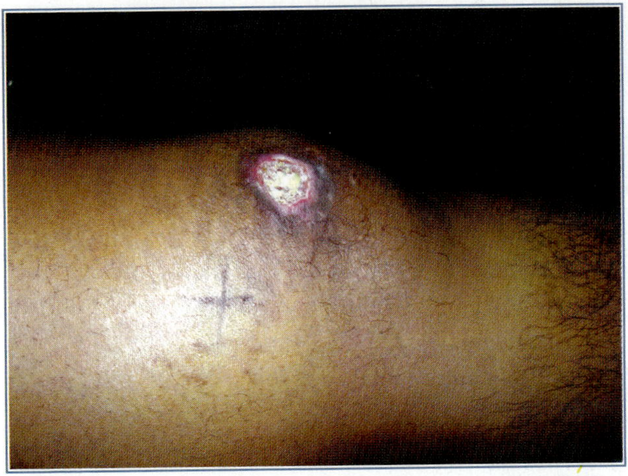

Fig 1.1: Wound over the anterior aspect of the knee joint due to fall. This has led to the development of traumatic synovitis. Note the fullness in the suprapatellar pouch. Mark the superomedial margin of the knee

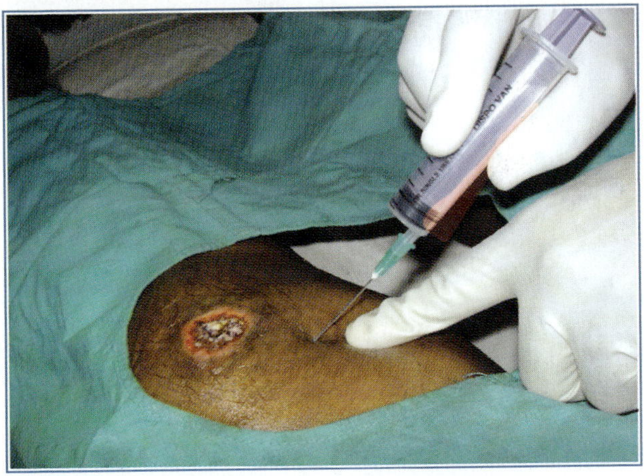

Fig. 1.2: Push the patella laterally and insert the needle through the point marked

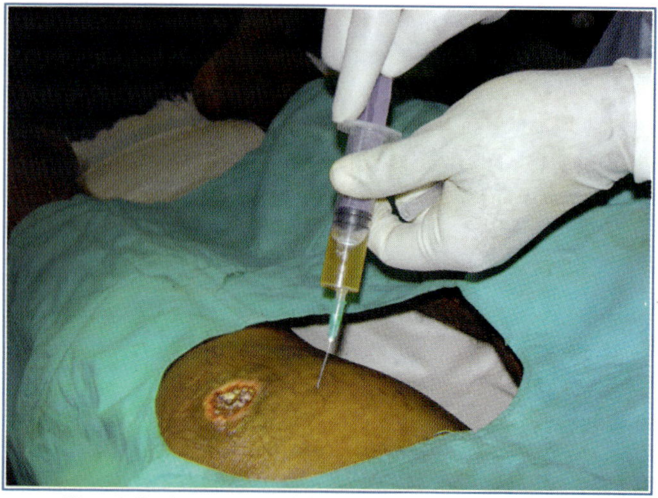

Fig. 1.3: Aspiration of the synovial fluid through an 18-gauge needle

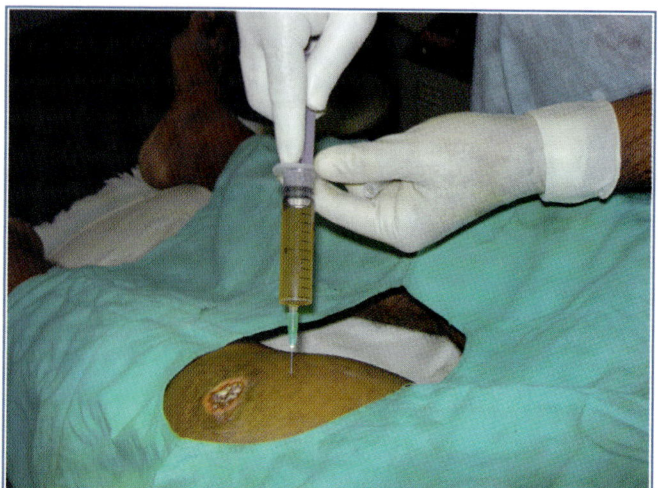

Fig. 1.4: Aspiration continued and the aspirate appears straw coloured indicating synovitis

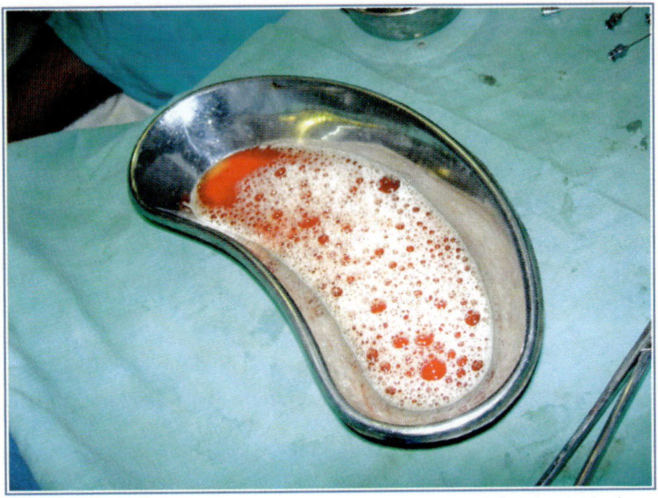

Fig 1.5: Collection of the blood tinged synovial fluid in a kidney tray. This confirms the diagnosis of traumatic synovitis. This has both therapeutic (pain relieved) and diagnostic (cause detected) value

Materials used: It is a mixture of a local anaesthetic preferably a 2 per cent plain lignocaine and a few cc of normal saline. While the first one alleviates the existing pain while the latter heightens it. But both indicate the course of origin of the unpleasant pain and thus indirectly help in making a diagnosis.

Diagnostic Injection Techniques

These have a wide role in identifying the source of pain in some soft tissue conditions and in low-backache conditions. The disappearance of pain after injecting local anaesthetic drug into the facets, nerve roots, foramen, disc, etc helps clearly establish the source of pain and with it the correct diagnosis.

Therapeutic Injection Techniques in Orthopaedics

As in diagnosis, so in therapeutics, injection techniques consists of joint aspirations and specific injection techniques.

a. *Therapeutic joint aspirations:* Therapeutic joint aspirations are sometimes necessary to remove blood, pus, large effusions, sinovial fluid, etc. (See Box).

Vital facts: Do you know the conditions requiring therapeutic joint aspirations? Well it is:

- Synovitis may be traumatic and nontraumatic
- Septic arthritis
- Haemarthrosis
- Acute large effusions
- Crystal synovitis
- Effusions that interfere with function

And do you know why it is necessary to remove these?

- Blood: As this acts as an irritant and causes synovitis
- Pus: As this activates the antibodies and causes joint destruction
- Large synovial effusions: As this causes stretching of the capsule, pain and loss of function.

b. *Therapeutic injections:* A lot many orthopaedic conditions affecting different joints and parts of the body can be treated by injections.

INDICATIONS

Injection treatment techniques are useful in the following conditions:

- Arthritis
- Synovitis
- Bursitis

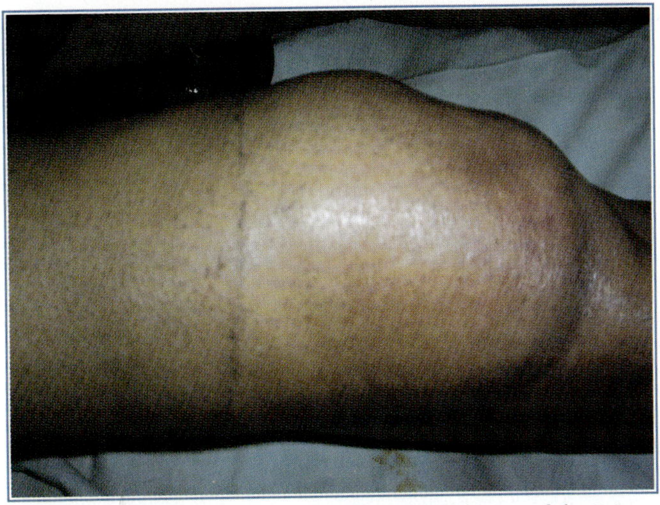

Fig. 1.6: Swelling of the knee joint within 2 hours of the injury suggests hemarthrosis

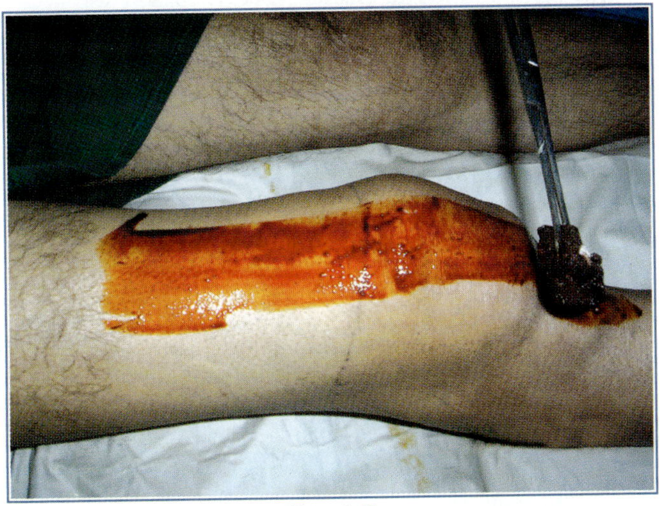

Fig. 1.7

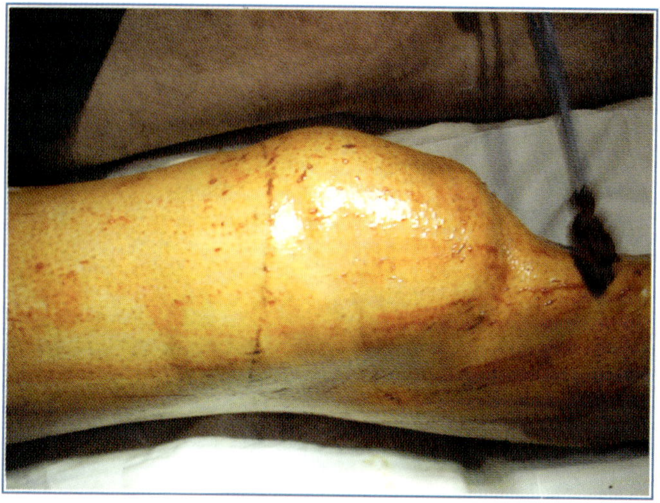

Fig. 1.8

Figs 1.7 and 1.8: The part is being painted with povidone-iodine

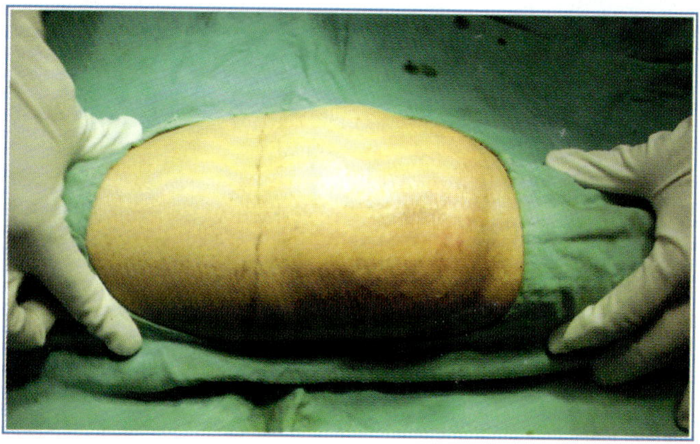

Fig. 1.9: The part is draped with a sterile towel

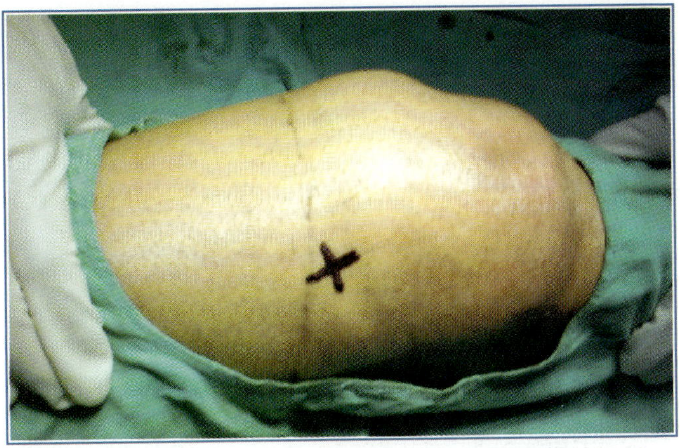

Fig. 1.10: Superolateral corner of the patella is marked with a sterile marker

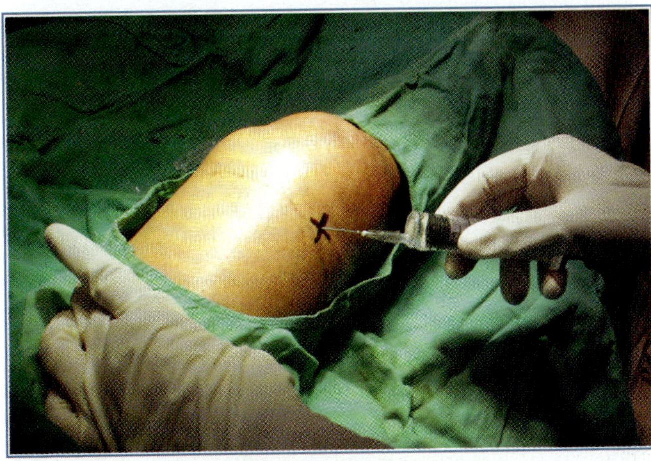

Fig. 1.11: Infiltration of the skin with 2 per cent plain local anaesthesia

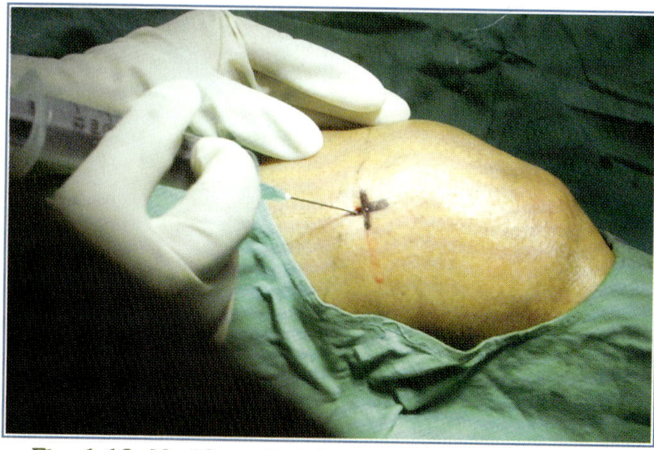

Fig. 1.12: No 18 needle is being introduced into the joint through the point marked

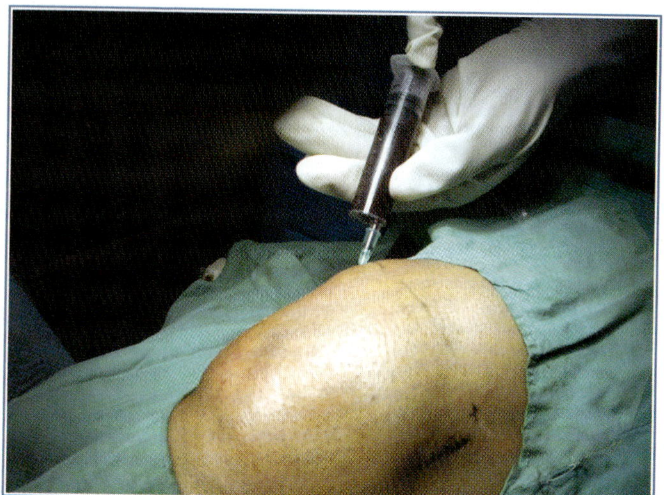

Fig. 1.13: Aspiration of dark colored blood

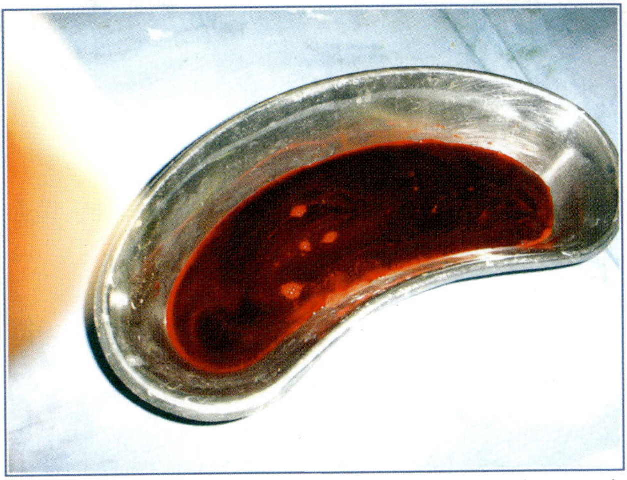

Fig. 1.14: Aspirated blood without fat globules indicating that the source of blood is from the torn ligaments and not from an intra-articular fracture within the knee

- Tendinitis
- Tenosynovitis
- Nodules
- Enthesopathies
- Trigger points
- Compression neuropathies like the compartmental syndrome, etc
- Crystal-induced arthritis: Gout, pseudogout, etc.

Quick facts: Arthritis and injection techniques:
- Rheumatoid arthritis – Commonest conditions requiring injection therapy
- Osteoarthritis
- Seronegative arthropathy:
- Ankylosing spondylitis
- Reiter's syndrome
- Psoriatic arthropathy.

Contraindications

- Overlying cellulitis
- Severe coagulopathy
- Anticoagulant therapy
- Septic effusion
- More than 3 injections per year in weight-bearing joints.
- Lack of response after 2 to 4 injections
- Bacteraemia
- Unstable joints
- Inaccesible joints
- Joint prosthesis
- Osteochondral fractures
- Overlying soft tissue infections or dermatitis

When does injection treatment make its grand entry as treatment modality in the field of orthopaedics?

- When peripheral joints are affected
- When two or more joints are actively inflamed and other joints are controlled by drugs
- In conditions mentioned previously
- When routine conservative measures fail to relieve pain as in Tennis elbow, golfer's elbow, low-backache, osteoarthritis, etc.

ABOUT DRUGS

- *Long-acting steroid preparation:* These are more useful in chronic diseases like osteoarthritis, rheumatoid arthritis, etc
- *Short-acting steroid preparation:* These are useful in soft tissue lesions like trigger point conditions, etc.

Note: If long-acting steroids are used for soft tissue lesions, it may cause atrophy of fat, subcutaneous tissue, skin, etc.

- Dosage: For larger joints: 50 mg of hydrocortisone acetate,40 mg of methylprednisolone and 20 mg of triamcinolone acetate
- For smaller joints half of these dose
- In a large joint like the knee adequate amounts of fluid is used along with the steroid to prevent it from remaining in one place

Choice of a needle:

- For very large effusions—19-gauge needle
- For injections without aspiration and for smaller joints like the interphalangeal joints, etc—23-gauge needle
- Widely used needles—23-gauge.

Materials Required for the Injection Techniques

- For skin preparation 1% chlorhexidine in spirit or a weak iodine solution
- A range of needles and syringes of different sizes
- Specimen sterile bottles to collect the aspirates
- Local anesthetics without adrenalin
- Steroids: hydrocortisone acetate (20 mg/ml), methylprednisolone acetate (40 mg/ml) and triamcinolone hexachloride
- Swab, dressings and gauge
- Elastocrepe bandages
- Saline to distend the joints
- Forceps for removing the jammed needles.

Note:

- *Strict asepsis or a non-touch technique and disposable syringes and needles are a must.*
- *Single dose ampoules are usually preferred*
- *Sterile towels, masks and gloves are often not required.*

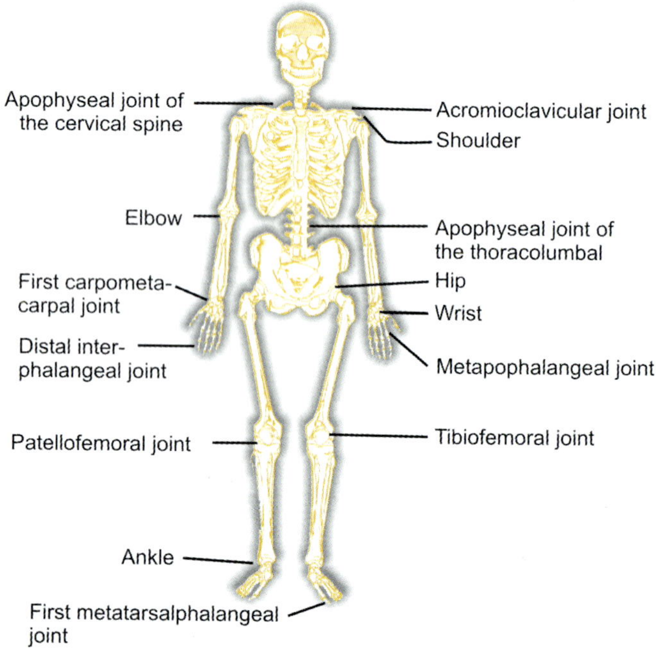

Fig. 1.15: Showing various joints in the body where injection techniques can be practiced both for therapeutic and diagnostic purposes

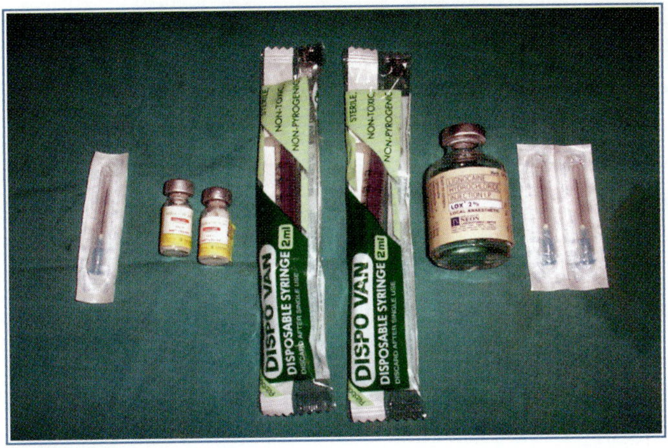

Fig. 1.16: Showing the materials required for injection in orthopaedics. Disposable syringes, 2 per cent lignocaine, steroid injection vials, sterile needles, etc

DO YOU KNOW THE MANTRAS FOR SUCCESS IN INJECTIONS?

a. *During the procedure*
   - Want first time success? Well, carefully palpate the bone landmarks and surfaces before injecting
   - Mark the site of injection with a marker or a thumbnail mark
   - It is better to approach the joint from the extensor surface to prevent damage to the important neuro-vascular structures lying on the flexor aspects
   - For skin preparation liberally apply chlorhexidine solution in spirit or weak iodine solution
   - For prolonged procedures like arthrography use towels.

To minimize the pre- and post-injection discomfort do the following:

- Infiltrate the skin with 1 to 2 per cent solution of lignocaine
- A local anaesthetic spray
- A quick insertion of the needle into the joint causes minimum pain. However, this requires practice and skill.

b. *About the patient*

- The patient should be relaxed because injection becomes difficult if the muscles are tensed
- The best position is supine with the head supported over a pillow. This is the ideal position to treat a vasovagal attack if encountered
- To position the limb correctly and to reassure the patient use the services of a nurse
- The patients who are going to benefit are those with warm swollen joints and with stiffness in the morning
- Those not likely to benefit are those with crepitus, severe X-ray changes or instability.

c. *Certain important precautions that needs to be observed for better results.*

- Do not give more than three injections in the same joint or area for fear of suppressing the inflammation and causing neuropathic joint due to the use of local anaesthetics
- Maintain a gap of one month between the injections
- Do not inject if there is a possibility of septic arthritis or sepsis elsewhere
- Aspirate before the injection to confirm no vessel

- While injecting into the soft tissues, jam the needle tightly as the contents have to be injected with force
- Warn the patient about the post-injection pain
- Instruct the patient to use the joint carefully for 24 hours after the injection
- The first injection is often the most successful
- The response in smaller joints is better and long lasting than the larger joints
- The maximum beneficial effects of an injection will be seen in the first few days itself
- Do not inject directly into the vessels, nerves, tendons etc.
- Avoid damaging the articular cartilage
- Limit to one large joint per visit.

Do You Know the Reasons for Failure of the Injections?

- Improper identification of the site
- Improper penetration
- Improper diagnosis
- Improper technique
- Improper drugs
- Improper dosage
- Improper person giving it.

Post-injection Advice and Follow-up

After the injection give the patients the following advice:

- Post-injection, the joint may remain painful for 24 hours
- The benefits of the injection may be seen several days later

- After the injection the joint needs to be rested for 1 to 2 days
- Avoid sports for at least 5 days
- No exercises for few days
- No heat therapy immediately after the injection.

Complications

- Post-injection flare (2-5%)
- Steroid arthropathy (0-8%)
- Tendon rupture (<1%)
- Facial flushing (<1%)
- Skin atrophy or depigmentations (<1%)
- Iatrogenic infectious arthritis
- Transient paraesis of injected extremity (rare)
- Hypersensitivity reaction
- Asymptomatic pericapsular calcification
- Hyperglycaemia in diabetes mellitus patients
- Acceleration of cartilage attrition

Before we begin let us try to get familiarized with certain basic requirements of drugs for injection techniques in the field of orthopaedics:

RECOMMENDED LOCAL ANAESTHETICS

Commonly Used Drugs

1. *Lignocaine also called lidocaine*
   - Dose: 3 mg/kg
   - Onset of action: Quick
   - Duration of action: 1 to 2 hours.

2. *Levobupivacaine*
    - Dose: 4 mg/kg
    - Onset of action: Slow
    - Duration of action: 2 to 4 hours.
3. *Bupivacaine*
    - Dose: 2 mg/kg
    - Onset of action: Slow
    - Duration of action: 2 to 4 hours.
4. *Ropivacaine*
    - Dose: 4 mg/kg
    - Onset of action: Fast
    - Duration of action: 2 to 4 hours.

RECOMMENDED CORTICOSTEROID INJECTIONS

1. Triamcinolone
    - Duration of action: 12 to 36 hours
    - Equivalent dosage: 4
    - Relative anti-inflammatory potency: 5
    - Relative mineralocorticoid potency: 0
2. Methylprednisolone
    - Duration of action: 12 to 36 hours
    - Equivalent dosage: 4
    - Relative anti-inflammatory potency: 5
    - Relative mineralocorticoid potency: 0.5
3. Dexamethasone
    - Duration of action: 48 hours
    - Equivalent dosage: 0.75
    - Relative anti-inflammatory potency: 25
    - Relative mineralocorticoid potency: 0

4. Hydrocortisone
   - Duration of action: 12
   - Equivalent dosage: 20
   - Relative anti-inflammatory potency: 1
   - Relative mineralocorticoid potency: 2

Note: Triamcinolone diacetate injections are best used for the spine.

Quick facts: Types of corticosteroids

A. *Short-acting/low potency*
   - Cortisone
   - Hydrocortisone

B. Intermediate acting/intermediate potency
   - Prednisone
   - Predinosolone tebutate (Hydeltra)
   - Triamcinolone (Aristocort, Aristospan, Kenalog)

D. Long-acting and high potency
   - Dexamethasone sodium phosphate (Decadron)
   - Betamethasone (Celestone soluspan).

Well Known Side Effects of Corticosteroids

A. General side effects
   - Arthropathy
   - Impaired glucose tolerance
   - Irregularity of the menstrual cycle
   - Myopathy and muscle wasting
   - Osteoporosis
   - Psychologic upset
   - Suppression of the adrenal function.

B. Local side effects
   - Depigmentation of the skin
   - Atrophy of the subcutaneous tissue

- Infection
- Rupture of the injected tendons.

RECOMMENDED NEEDLES

1. Joint injection: Needle gauges 22-25 with length of 1.5 inches.
2. Joint aspiration: Needle gauges 18-20 with length of 1.5 inches.
3. Special circumstances: Spinal needle.

e.g.

a. Obesity: interferes with joint or bursa access
b. Trochanteric/bursitis.

RECOMMENDED NEUROLYTIC AGENTS

- Aqueous phenol 6 per cent
- 100 per cent alcohol diluted to 50 per cent

RECOMMENDED RESUSCITATION DRUGS

1. Atropine
    - Recommended dosage: 0.2 to 0.4 mg
    - Indication: Bradycardia due to vagal dominance.
2. Ephedrine
    - Recommended dosage: 5 to 10 mg
    - Indication: Hypotension due to sympathetic block.
3. Lignocaine
    - Recommended dosage: 50 to 100 mg iv bolus
    - Indication: Ventricular arrhythmias.

4. Midazolam
   - Recommended dosage: 1 to 3 mg iv increments
   - Indication: Seizures due to local anaesthetics.
5. Diazepam
   - Recommended dosage: 2.5 to 5 mg iv increments
   - Indication: Seizures due to local anaesthetics.
6. Thiopental
   - Recommended dosage: 50 to 100 mg iv increments
   - Indication: Seizures due to local anaesthetics.
7. Succinylcholine
   - Recommended dosage: 50 to 100 mg iv bolus
   - Indication: Muscle relaxation airway control.

Note: A full range of drugs necessary for ACLS (Advanced Cardiac Life Support) with prefilled syringes should be made available in the operating room.

RECOMENDED RESUSCITATION EQUIPMENT

- Oxygen cylinders
- Endotracheal tubes of different sizes
- Magill's forceps
- Full range—oro and nasopharangeal airways
- Full range—laryngoscopes and blades
- Full range masks and bags
- Breathing system for positive pressure ventilation.

Now, let us try to know the injection procedures for individual joints and other conditions is a systematic manner.

Section 2

Injection Techniques in the Upper Limbs

SHOULDER COMPLEX

INTRA-ARTICULAR INJECTIONS

Shoulder Joint

Indications

- Osteoarthritis
- Rheumatoid arthritis
- Posttraumatic arthritis
- Rotator cuff arthropathy.

Less Common

- Infection
- Collagen vascular disease
- Villonodular synovitis
- Lyme's disease.

Presentation of Common Shoulder Conditions

- Pain is localized around the shoulder and upper arm
- Activity increases the pain
- Rest relieves the pain
- Pain is continuous in nature
- Pain interferes with sleep
- Popping sensation could be heard.

Clinical Signs

- Tenderness is present over the shoulder
- Crepitus
- Decreased range of motion exercises
- Muscle wasting.

Functional

- Simple day to day activities like combing the hair, buttoning a shirt, etc. may be affected.

Investigations

- Laboratory tests: This includes complete blood count, RA test, ESR, etc
- Plain X-ray of the shoulder joint
- MRI Scan very useful in rotator cuff injuries.

TECHNIQUES OF VARIOUS APPROACHES

Three approaches are described with respect to the shoulder joint:

- Anterior approach
- Posterior approach
- Lateral approach.

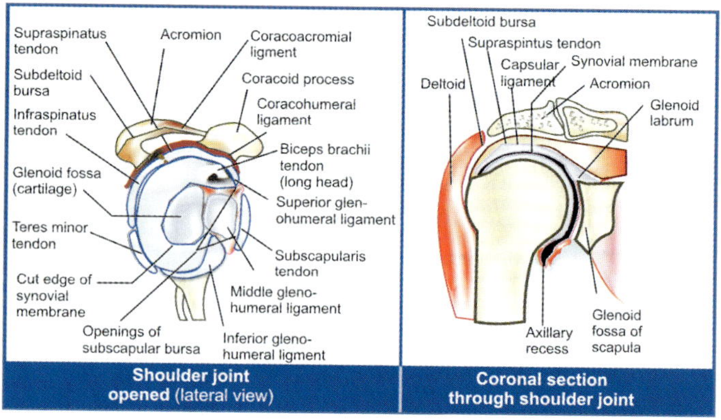

Fig. 2.1: Shoulder joint anatomy: Lateral and coronal views

Lateral Approach

- Position is sitting or supine
- Preparation is by painting the shoulder, subacromial and axillary regions with antiseptic solution
- Drape the area.

Injection Preparation

- Drugs: 0.25 per cent bupivacaine and 40 mg of methyl-prednisolone
- Quantity: 2 ml
- Syringe: 5 ml/1 ½ " in length/25-gauge needle.

Procedures

- Patient is put in the above position
- Identify the midpoint of the acromion
- Next locate the shoulder joint space which is about 2.5 cm below the midpoint
- Advance the needle carefully into this space
- If no resistance is felt, you are inside the joint
- If resistance is felt it means you have hit the bone Withdraw the needle redirect it more superiorly and medially
- Now slightly withdraw the piston of the syringe and inject the contents into the space
- If no resistance is felt, the injection is successful. If you feel resistance, the needle could be in the ligament or

tendon. Now advance the needle slightly further and inject again
- Apply sterile pressure dressing
- Ice packs helps.

Complications

- Infection
- Transient increase in pain (seen in 25%)
- Rashes
- Haematoma.

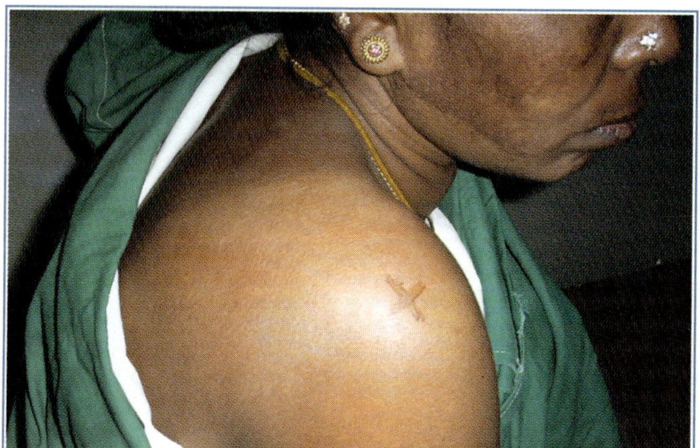

Fig. 2.2A: Mark the midpoint of the lateral edge of the acromion

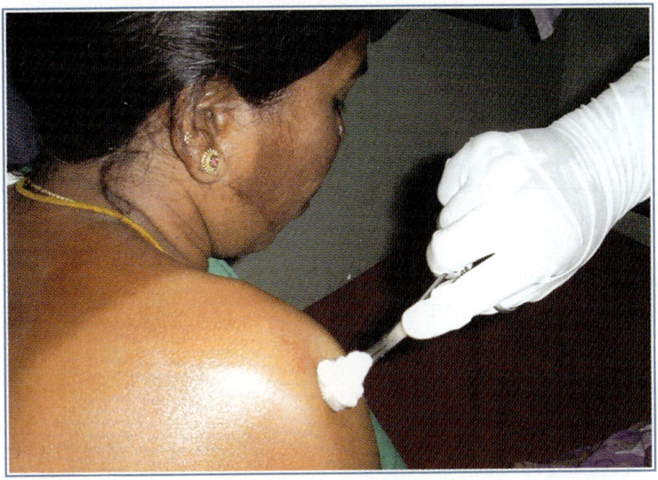

Fig. 2.2B: Now paint the area with antiseptic solution

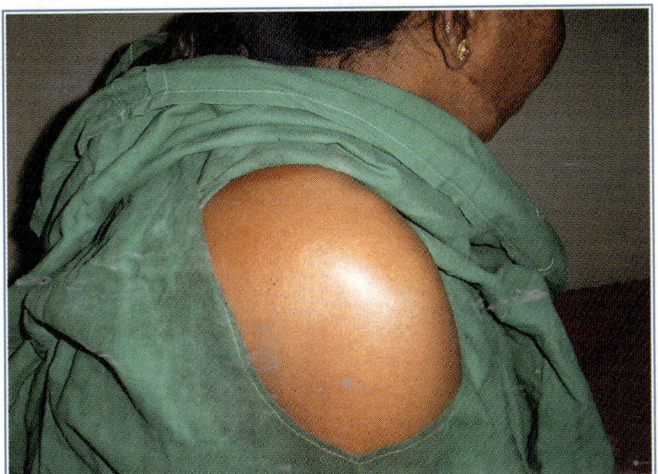

Fig. 2.2C: Drape the area

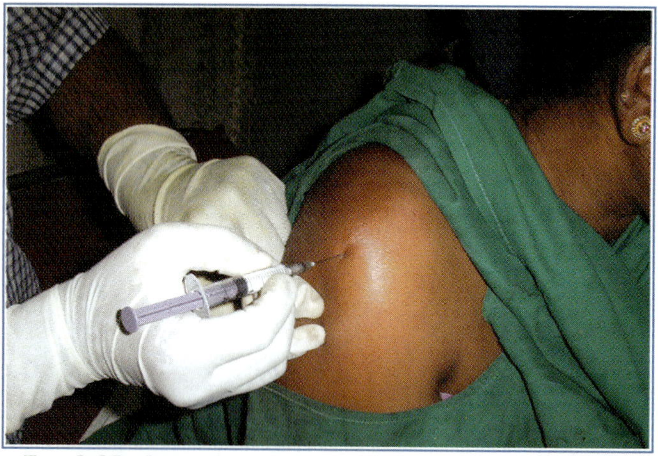

Fig. 2.2D: Insert the needle at the point marked previously

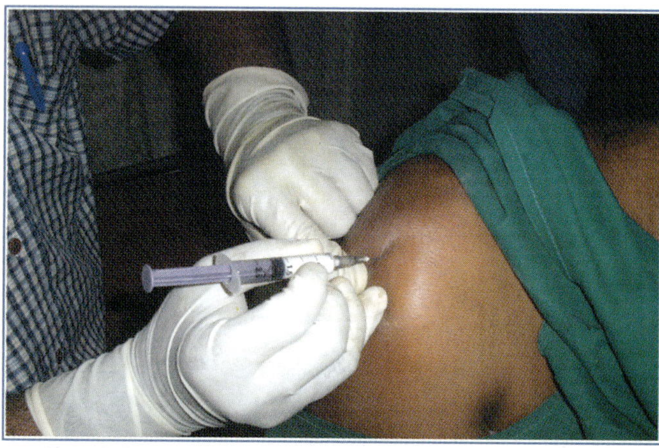

Fig. 2.2E: Manipulate gently and proceed beneath the acromion

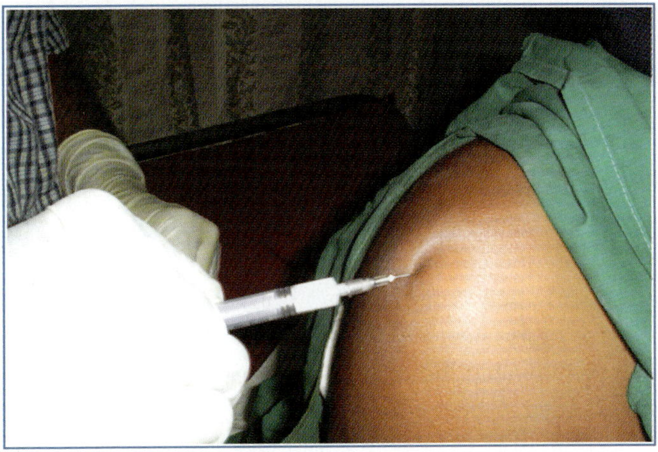

Fig. 2.2F: Slowly inject the contents of the syringe

After Care

- Simple analgesics
- A course of antibiotics
- Local heat and range of motion exercises—after several days
- Avoid vigorous exercises.

Advantages

This is the best approach for supraspinatus tendinitis.

Posterior Approach

Advantages: This approach is useful when one is unsure about the diagnosis and can be employed for lesions of the supraspinatus, infraspinatus, and subscapularis tendons and in the disorders of the glenohumeral joints.

Procedures

- Patient sits with the back to the doctor with arm by the sides and shoulder externally rotated
- Palpate the spine of the scapula and run the finger along till it turns forward to form the acromion process at the posterolateral corner
- Palpate the coracoid process with the forefinger
- The line between these two bony processes forms the track of the needle
- Now advance the needle into the upper recess of the shoulder 1" below the acromion. You are successful if you are able to inject without resistance.

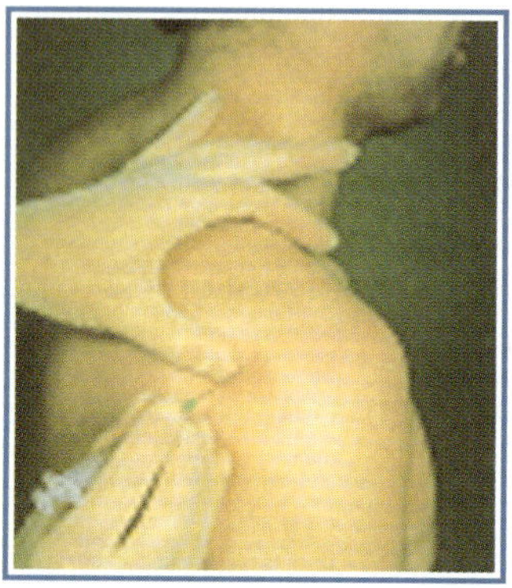

Fig. 2.3: Posterior approach of injection technique into shoulder joint

Anterior Approach

Position: Patient can sit or lie on the back with the forearm placed on the abdomen and the shoulder is partially internally rotated.

Procedures

- Identify the head of the humerus by passive rotation
- Now feel for the coracoid process
- Pass the needle in the direction of the joint line directed posteriorly just lateral (about 1 cm) to the coracoid process and inject

Disadvantages: This approach is technically demanding

After care: At the injection site, after the injection
- Apply icepacks
- Apply a firm sterile bandage under pressure.

Complications

- Infection (hence follow strict aseptic measures)
- Transient increase of pain (seen in 25% of the cases)
- Ecchymosis
- Haematoma formation.

Note: The incidence of ecchymosis and haematoma formation can be reduced if immediately after the injection, a firm sterile pressure bandage is applied.

Vital facts: Strictly observe the following after the injection:
- Simple analgesics and NSAIDs are advised
- To prevent the exacerbation of pain, avoid heat and gentle range of motion exercises for few days
- Avoid vigorous exercises for few days to prevent increase in pain.

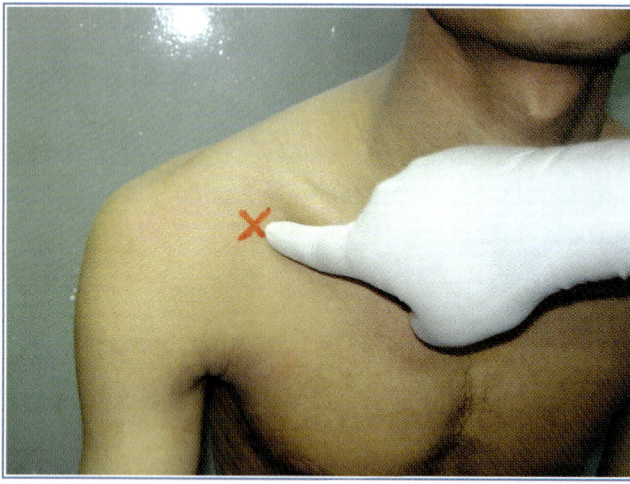

Fig. 2.4A: Feel and mark the coracoid process with a sterile marker

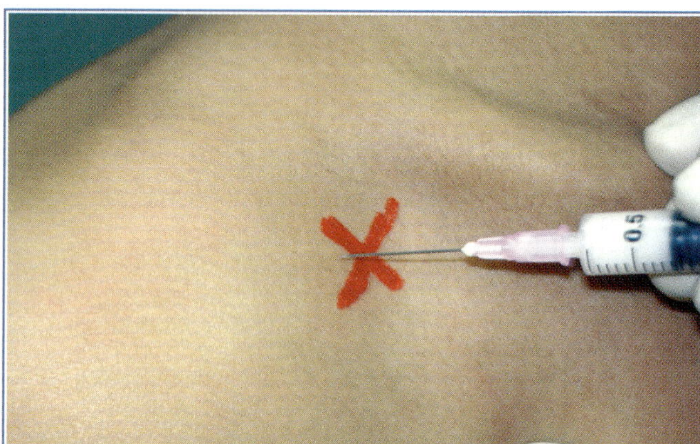

Fig. 2.4B: Pass the needle in the direction of the joint line directed posteriorly and lateral to the coracoid process and inject

The Acromioclavicular Joint

Indications

- Acute trauma
- Repeated strain due to throwing injuries
- Arthritis of the ACM joint.

Presentation

- Pain on reaching across the chest
- Inability to sleep on the affected shoulder
- Grinding sensation on first awakening.

Signs

- Swelling present
- Tenderness is present
- Downward traction increases the pain
- Passive abduction increases the pain
- Joint instability if ligaments are ruptured.

Investigations

- Plain X-ray: reveals narrowing of the joint space and sclerosis
- MRI: Useful if the ligament rupture is suspected.

Procedures

Position

Supine or sitting. The arm is resting by the side and the shoulder is externally rotated.

Preparation

- Paint the area in and around the shoulder with antiseptic solution
- Drape the area.

Injection Preparation

- Drugs: 0.25 per cent preservative free bupivacaine and 40 mg of methylprednisolone
- Quantity: 0.5 ml to 1 ml (due to limited capacity of the joint)
- Syringe: 1 ½" with 25-gauge needle.

Techniques

- Identify the top of the acromion with careful palpation
- Locate the ACM joint space which lies 1 inch medial to the above point seen as a slight depression where clavicle meets acromion.
- Insert needle from anterior and superior approach
- Advance the needle at an angle of 20 degrees medially into the joint and slowly inject the drug
- If you hit the bone, withdraw the needle slightly and redirect it more medially.

Resistance vs Inference

- If no resistance is felt, there could be disruption of joint space due to torn ligaments, MRI is suggested

- If significant resistance is felt, the needle could be in the ligament or tendon. Withdraw or advance slightly and re-inject
- If some resistance is felt, congratulations, you are in the right space as the joint is small and the capsule is dense.

After Care

At the injection site, after the injection

- Apply icepacks
- Apply a firm sterile bandage under pressure.

Complications

- Infection (hence follow strict aseptic measures)
- Transient increase of pain (seen in 25% of the cases)

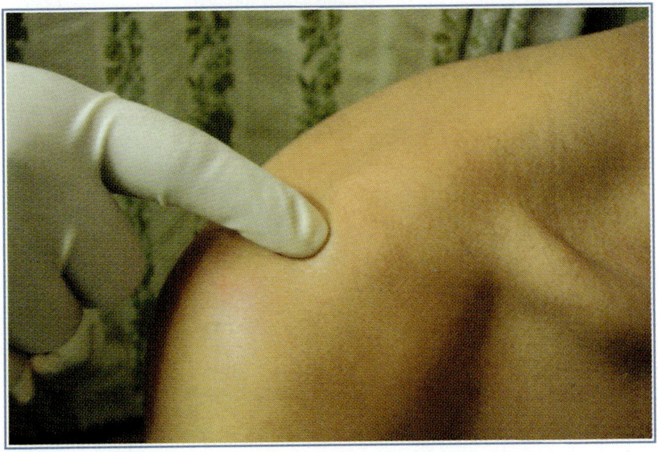

Fig. 2.5A: Identify the top of the acromion

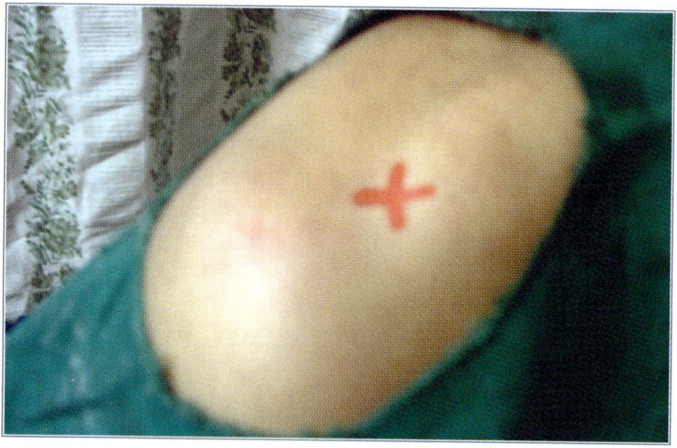

Fig. 2.5B: Mark it with a sterile markter

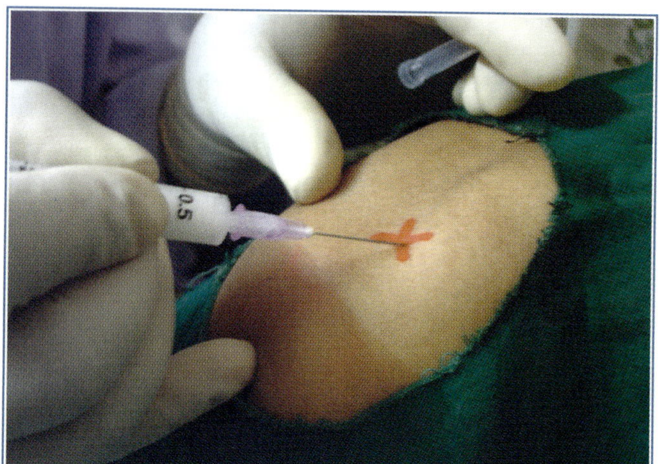

Fig. 2.5C: Advance the needle at an angle of 20 degrees medially into the joint

- Ecchymosis
- Haematoma formation.

Note: The incidence of ecchymosis and haematoma formation can be reduced if immediately after the injection, a firm sterile pressure bandage is applied.

Vital facts: Strictly observe the following after the injection:
- Simple analgesics and NSAIDs are advised
- To prevent the exacerbation of pain, avoid heat and gentle range of motion exercises for few days
- Avoid vigorous exercises for few days to prevent increase in pain.

THE STERNOCLAVICULAR JOINTS

Indications

Common

- Osteoarthritis
- Injuries
- Rheumatoid arthritis
- Overuse.

Uncommon

- Ankylosing spondylitis
- Reiter's syndrome
- Psoriatic arthritis
- Tumour invasion, e.g. thymoma
- Metastasis.

Presentation

- Patient complains of pain and sometimes it mimics the pain of cardiac origin
- Pain is reproduced by active protraction or retraction of the shoulder
- Pain increases on elevation of the shoulder
- Shrugging of the shoulder increases the pain
- Complaints of clicking sensation with movement
- There could be swelling and tenderness.

Investigations

- Laboratory tests: This consists of CBC, ESR, PSA, ANA tests
- Plain X-ray to rule out occult bony pathology
- MRI: If joint instability is suspected.

Procedures

Position: Supine or sitting

Preparation

- Paint the area in and around the sternoclavicular with antiseptic solution
- Drape the area.

Injection Preparation

- Drugs: 0.25 per cent preservative free bupivacaine and 40 mg of methylprednisolone

- Quantity: 0.5 ml to 1 ml (due to limited capacity of the joint)
- Syringe: 1 ½" with 25-gauge needle.

Techniques

- Identify the sternal end of the clavicle with careful palpation
- Slight indentation at the point where clavicle meets the manubrium sternum is the sternoclavicular joint space
- Advance the needle at an angle of 45 degrees medially into the joint and slowly inject the drug
- If you hit the bone, withdraw the needle slightly and redirect it more medially.

Resistance vs Inference

- If no resistance is felt, joint space is missed
- If significant resistance is felt, the needle could be in the ligament or tendon. Withdraw or advance slightly and re-inject
- If some resistance is felt, congratulations, you are in the right space as the joint is small and the capsule is dense.

After Care

At the injection site, after the injection

- Apply icepacks
- Apply a firm sterile bandage under pressure.

Complications

- Infection (hence follow strict aseptic measures)
- Transient increase of pain (seen in 25% of the cases)
- Ecchymosis
- Haematoma formation.

Note: The incidence of ecchymosis and haematoma formation can be reduced if immediately after the injection, a firm sterile pressure bandage is applied.

Vital facts: Strictly observe the following after the injection:

- Simple analgesics and NSAIDs are advised
- To prevent the exacerbation of pain, avoid heat and gentle range of motion exercises for few days
- Avoid vigorous exercises for few days to prevent increase in pain.

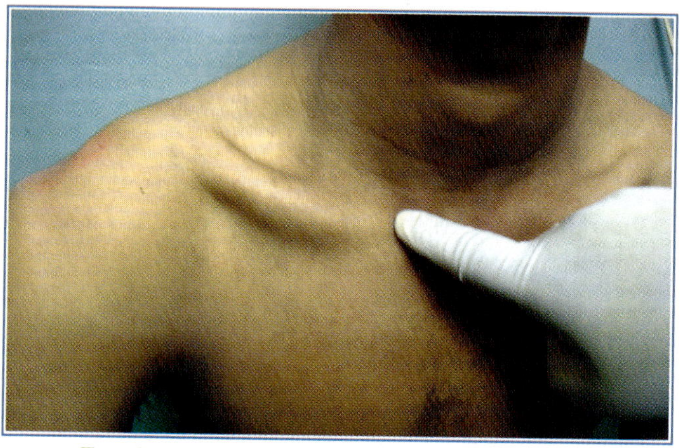

Fig. 2.6A: Identify the sternal end of the clavicle

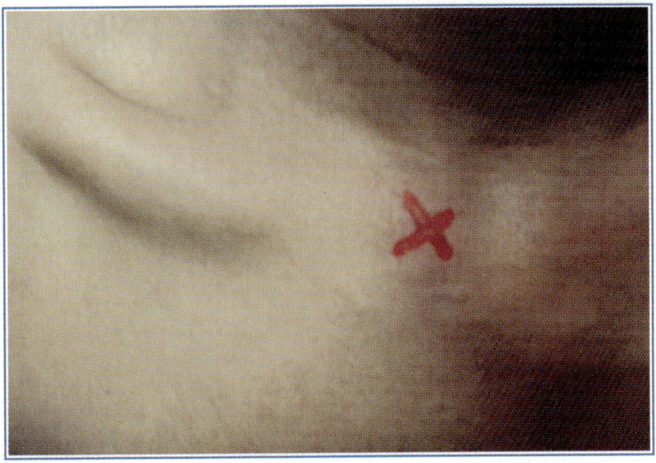

Fig. 2.6B: Slight indentation at the point where the clavicle meets the manubrium sternum is the sternoclavicular joint. Mark it with a sterile marker

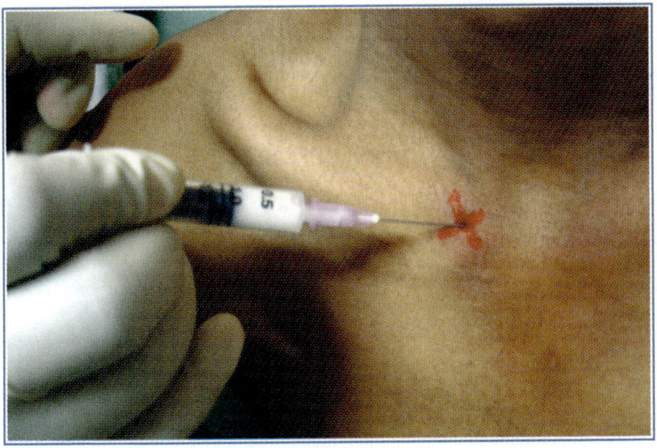

Fig. 2.6C: Advance the needle at an angle of 45-degree medially into the joint

LOCAL INFILTRATION OF THE INJECTIONS

Infraspinatus Tendinitis

Indications

It is due to repeated overuse or misuse.

Presentations

- Pain is constant, severe and localised to the deltoid region
- Significant disturbance in sleep
- Pain increases on lateral rotation and abduction
- Patient keeps the scapula rotated anteriorly to remove tension from the tendon
- Progressive decrease in shoulder range of movements
- Simple day to day activities are affected.

Late Features

- Muscle wasting
- Frozen shoulder.

Investigations

- Laboratory tests: CBC, ESR, ANA, etc
- Plain X-ray of the shoulder
- MRI if ligament rupture is suspected.

Procedures

- Position: Sitting with arm supported on a table and elbow flexed to 90 degrees

- Preparation: Paint the shoulder with antiseptic solution
- Drape the area.

Injection Preparation

- Drugs: 0.25 per cent preservative free bupivacaine and 40 mg of methylprednisolone
- Quantity: 0.5 ml to 1 ml (due to limited capacity of the joint)
- Syringe: 1 ½" with 25-gauge needle.

Techniques

- In the above position, rotate the arm externally. This brings the insertion of the infraspinatus muscle out from the deltoid muscle
- Identify the posterior angle of the acromion and the lateral epicondyle
- The insertion of the infraspinatus tendon lies in a direct line with the lateral epicondyle approximately 45 degrees inferior to the posterior angle of the acromion. Mark this point with a sterile marker
- Advance the needle at this point till it hits the bone
- Now gently withdraw the needle slightly and inject the drug.

Resistance vs Inference

- If no resistance is felt, needle could be in the joint space or the tendon could be ruptured
- If significant resistance is felt, the needle could be in the ligament or tendon. Withdraw or advance slightly and re-inject

- If some resistance is felt, congratulations, you are in the right space as the joint is small and the capsule is dense.

After Care

At the injection site, after the injection

- Apply icepacks
- Apply a firm sterile bandage under pressure.

Complications

- Infection (hence follow strict aseptic measures)
- Transient increase of pain (seen in 25% of the cases)
- Ecchymosis
- Haematoma formation.

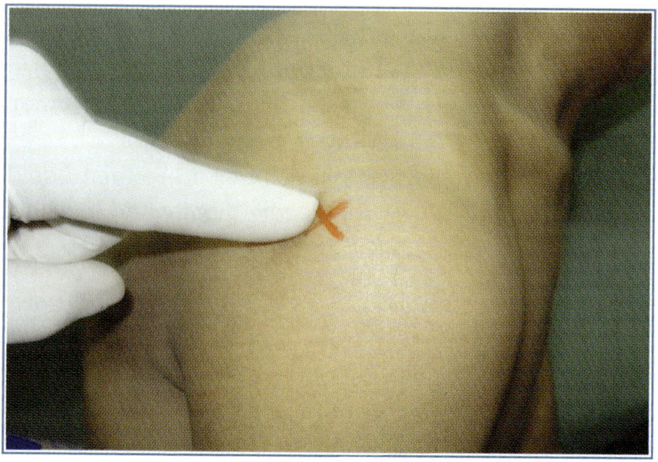

Fig. 2.7A: Identify the posterior angle of the acromion. Mark it with a sterile marker

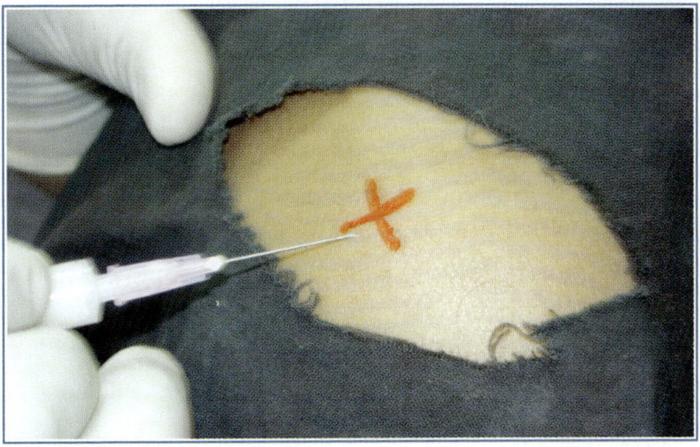

Fig. 2.7B: Advance the needle at an angle of 45 degrees inferior to the posterior angle of the acromion

Note: The incidence of ecchymosis and haematoma formation can be reduced if immediately after the injection, a firm sterile pressure bandage is applied.

Vital facts: Strictly observe the following after the injection:
- Simple analgesics and NSAIDs are advised
- To prevent the exacerbation of pain, avoid heat and gentle range of motion exercises for few days
- Avoid vigorous exercises for few days to prevent increase in pain.

Supraspinatus Tendinitis

Indications

- Due to repeated overuse or misuse of the shoulder
- Due to carrying heavy loads in front and away from the body
- Due to vigorous use of the exercise equipment.

Presentations

- Pain is constant and severe in nature. Sleep is often affected
- Shrugging appearance, this is due to elevation of the scapula to protect the inflamed tendon
- Positive Dawbarn's sign: Here there is tenderness over the greater tuberosity with the arm hanging down and on fully abducting the arm it disappears
- Progressive decrease in the range of motion
- Simple day to day activities are affected.

Late Features

- Muscle wasting
- Frozen shoulder.

Investigations

- Laboratory tests: CBC, ESR, ANA, etc
- Plain X-ray of the shoulder
- MRI if ligament rupture is suspected.

Procedures

- Position: Sitting or supine with forearm medially rotated behind the back

  Caution: However beware of the vasovagal attack in the sitting position
- Preparation: Paint the shoulder with antiseptic solution
- Drape the area.

Injection Preparation

- Drugs: 0.25 per cent preservative free bupivacaine and 40 mg of methylprednisolone
- Quantity: 0.5 ml to 1 ml (due to limited capacity of the joint)
- Syringe: 1 ½" with 25-gauge needle.

Techniques

- In the above position, identify the lateral epicondyle
- Now trace the humerus superiorly up to the anterior edge of the acromion
- Just below this there is a slight indentation, which indicates the point of insertion of the supraspinatus tendon into the upper facet of the greater tuberosity. Mark this point with a sterile marker.
- Paint the area in and around the shoulder with an antiseptic lotion
- Reidentify the marked point above with a gloved finger
- Advance the needle perpendicular to this point till it hits the bone
- Now gently withdraw the needle slightly and inject the drug.

Reistance vs Inference

- If no resistance is felt, needle could be in the joint space or the tendon could be ruptured
- If significant resistance is felt, the needle could be in the ligament or tendon. Withdraw or advance slightly and re-inject

- If some resistance is felt, congratulations, you are in the right space as the joint is small and the capsule is dense.

After Care

At the injection site, after the injection

- Apply icepacks
- Apply a firm sterile bandage under pressure.

Complications

- Infection (hence follow strict aseptic measures)
- Transient increase of pain (seen in 25% of the cases)
- Ecchymosis
- Haematoma formation.

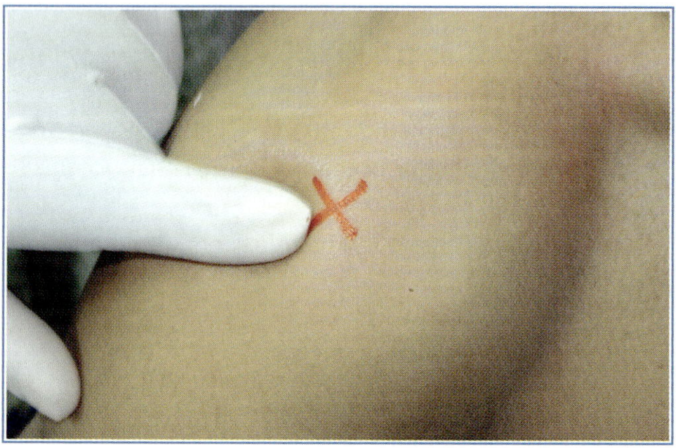

Fig. 2.8A: Identify the anterior edge of the acromion. Slight indentation below it indicates the point of insertion of the supraspinatus tendon. Mark it with a sterile marker

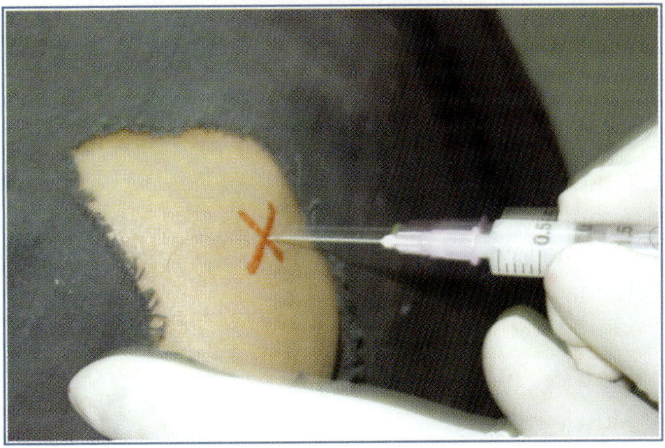

Fig. 2.8B: Advance the needle perpendicularly at this point

Note: The incidence of ecchymosis and haematoma formation can be reduced if immediately after the injection, a firm sterile pressure bandage is applied.

Vital facts: Strictly observe the following after the injection:
- Simple analgesics and NSAIDs are advised
- To prevent the exacerbation of pain, avoid heat and gentle range of motion exercises for few days
- Avoid vigorous exercises for few days to prevent increase in pain.

Subscapularis Tendinitis

Aetiology

- Due to repeated overuse or misuse
- Due to activities that require repeated adduction and medial rotation of the humerus as in repetitive motions during assembly line work.

Presentation

- Pain is constant and severe
- Significant sleep disturbance is noted
- Pain is localized in the anterior deltoid and shoulder
- Pain increases on resisted medial rotation active rotation and adduction
- Patient loathes to perform medial rotation of the humerus.

Late Features

- Muscle wasting
- Frozen shoulder.

Investigations

- Laboratory tests: CBC, ESR, ANA, etc
- Plain X-ray of the shoulder
- MRI if ligament rupture is suspected.

Procedures

- Position: Supine with the arm rotated externally by 45 degrees
- Preparation: Paint the shoulder with antiseptic solution
- Drape the area.

Injection Preparation

- Drugs: 0.25 per cent preservative free bupivacaine and 40 mg of methylprednisolone

- Quantity: 0.5 ml to 1 ml (Due to limited capacity of the joint)
- Syringe: 1 ½" with 25-gauge needle.

Techniques

- In the above position, identify the coracoid process anteriorly
- The lesser tuberosity lies just lateral to the coracoid process at which the tendon gets inserted.

Note: By passively rotating the arm, the lesser tuberosity can be easily palpated.

- Mark this point with a sterile marker
- Paint and drape the area
- Reidentify the point marked above with a gloved finger
- Advance the needle straight at this point till it hits the bone
- Now gently withdraw the needle slightly and inject the drug.

Resistance cs Inference

- If no resistance is felt, needle could be in the joint space or the tendon could be ruptured
- If significant resistance is felt, the needle could be in the ligament or tendon. Withdraw or advance slightly and re-inject
- If some resistance is felt, congratulations, you are in the right space as the joint is small and the capsule is dense.

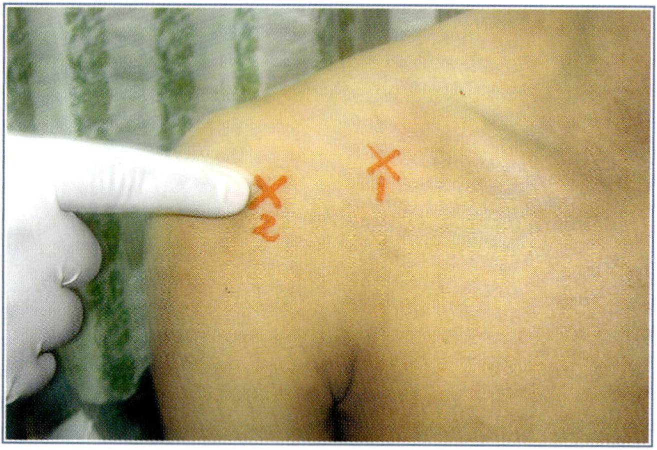

Fig. 2.9A: Identify the coracoid process and mark it as 1. Next identify the lesser tuberosity which lies one inch lateral to the coracoid process and mark it as 2

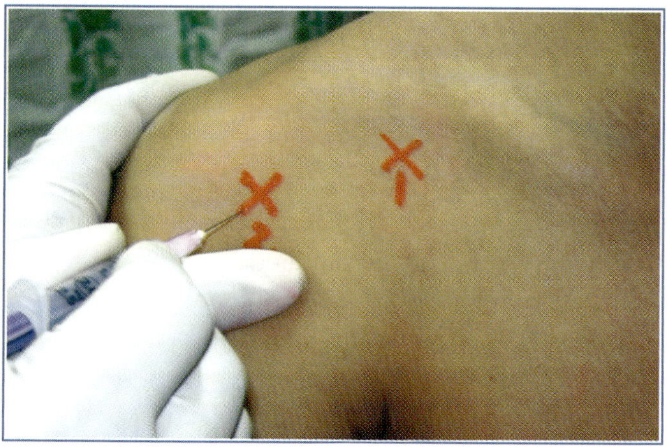

Fig. 2.9B: Advance the needle straight at the joint of mark 2

After Care

At the injection site, after the injection

- Apply icepacks
- Apply a firm sterile bandage under pressure.

Complications

- Infection (hence follow strict aseptic measures)
- Transient increase of pain (seen in 25% of the cases)
- Ecchymosis
- Haematoma formation.

Note: The incidence of ecchymosis and haematoma formation can be reduced if immediately after the injection, a firm sterile pressure bandage is applied.

Vital facts: Strictly observe the following after the injection:
- Simple analgesics and NSAIDs are advised
- To prevent the exacerbation of pain, avoid heat and gentle range of motion exercises for few days
- Avoid vigorous exercises for few days to prevent increase in pain.

Bicipital Tendinitis

Aetiology

- Overuse or misuse of the shoulder
- Attempting to start a recalcitrant lawn mover
- Practicing an overhead tennis serve
- Overaggressive follow through when driving golf balls.

Presentation

- Pain is constant, severe and localized anterioirly in the bicipital groove
- There could be complaints of catching sensation
- Attitude: Patient keeps the upper arm internally rotated
- Yergason's sign: Reproduction of pain on active supination of the forearm against resistance with the elbow flexed to 90 degrees.

Late Features

- Muscle wasting
- Frozen shoulder.

Investigations

- Laboratory tests: CBC, ESR, ANA, etc
- Plain X-ray of the shoulder
- MRI if ligament rupture is suspected.

Procedures

- Position: Supine with the arm by the side and shoulder rotated externally by 45 degrees
- Preparation: Paint the shoulder with antiseptic solution
- Drape the area.

Injection Preparation

- Drugs: 0.25 per cent preservative free bupivacaine and 40 mg of methylprednisolone
- Quantity: 0.5 ml to 1 ml (due to limited capacity of the joint)
- Syringe: 1 to 1 ½" with 25- to 27-gauge needle.

Techniques

- In the above position, identify the coracoid process anteriorly
- The lesser tuberosity lies just lateral to the coracoid process at which the tendon gets inserted.

Note: By passively rotating the arm, the lesser tuberosity can be easily palpated.

- Identify bicipital tendon in bicipital groove and locate the point of maximum tenderness
- Mark this point with a sterile marker
- Paint and drape the area
- Reidentify the point marked above with a gloved finger
- Advance the needle straight at this point parallel to bicipital groove till it hits the bone
- Needle should enter skin at 30°
- Now gently withdraw the needle slightly and inject the drug.

Resistance vs Inference

- If no resistance is felt, needle could be in the joint space or the tendon could be ruptured
- If significant resistance is felt, the needle could be in the ligament or tendon. Withdraw or advance slightly and re-inject
- If some resistance is felt, congratulations, you are in the right space as the joint is small and the capsule is dense.

Caution: Do not inject into bicipital tendon.

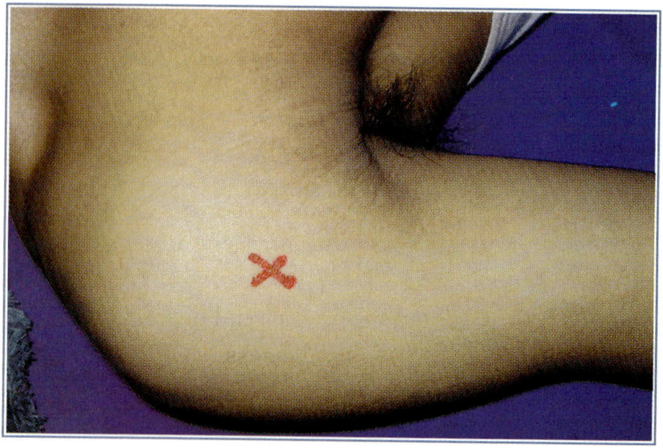

Fig. 2.10A: Identify the bicipital tendon in the bicipital groove and mark it

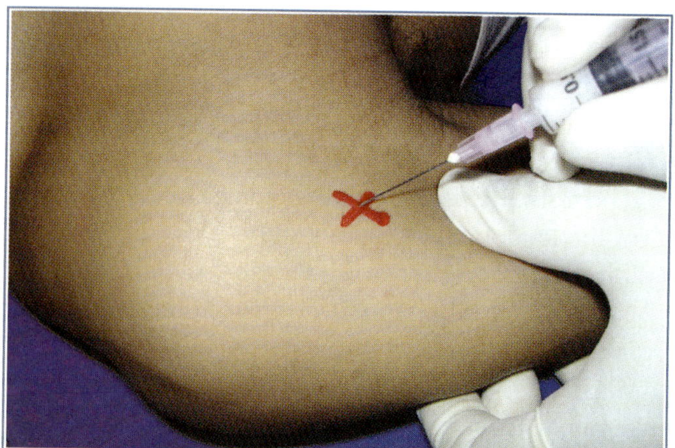

Fig. 2.10B: Insert the needle in a 30-degree cephalad direction at the marked point

After Care

At the injection site, after the injection

- Apply icepacks
- Apply a firm sterile bandage under pressure.

Complications

- Infection (hence follow strict aseptic measures)
- Transient increase of pain (seen in 25% of the cases)
- Ecchymosis
- Haematoma formation
- Rupture of bicipital tendon

Note: The incidence of ecchymosis and haematoma formation can be reduced if immediately after the injection, a firm sterile pressure bandage is applied.

Vital facts: Strictly observe the following after the injection:
- Simple analgesics and NSAIDs are advised
- To prevent the exacerbation of pain, avoid heat and gentle range of motion exercises for few days
- Avoid vigorous exercises for few days to prevent increase in pain.

Rotator Cuff Tear Pain

Aetiology

- Due to acute trauma
- Due to degeneration: This is more common and is seen in elderly patients.

Presentation

- Pain is constant and severe
- The tear could be partial or complete
- Inability to lift the affected arm above the level of the shoulder without using the other arm to lift it
- If the infraspinatus is involved patient has weakness on external rotation and if the supraspinatus is involved patient complains of weakness in abduction above the shoulder level
- Tenderness in the subacromial region
- Patient complains of inability to reach above the level of the shoulder in complete tears
- Drop arm test is positive
- Moseley's test: Instruct the patient to abduct the arm up to 90 degrees. Now add gentle resistance. This will force the arm to drop if there is complete tear
- Active ROM of the shoulder is affected but passive ROM is normal.

Late Features

- Muscle wasting
- Frozen shoulder.

Investigations

- Laboratory tests: CBC, ESR, ANA, etc
- Plain X-ray of the shoulder
- MRI if ligament rupture is suspected.

Procedures

- Position: Supine
- Preparation: Paint the shoulder with antiseptic solution
- Drape the area.

Injection Preparation

- Drugs: 0.25 per cent preservative free bupivacaine and 40 mg of methylprednisolone
- Quantity: 4 ml (due to limited capacity of the joint)
- Syringe: 5 ml /1 ½" with 25-gauge needle.

Techniques

- In the above position, identify the lateral edge of the acromion
- Mark the midpoint of the lateral edge of the acromion with a sterile marker. This is the injection site
- Paint and drape the area
- Reidentify the point marked above with a gloved finger
- Advance the needle under the acromion process in a cephalad direction directing it towards the opposite nipple.
- If you hit the bone, withdraw and redirect the needle slightly inferiorly and inject the drug.

Resistance vs Inference

- If no resistance is felt, needle could be in the joint space or the tendon could be ruptured

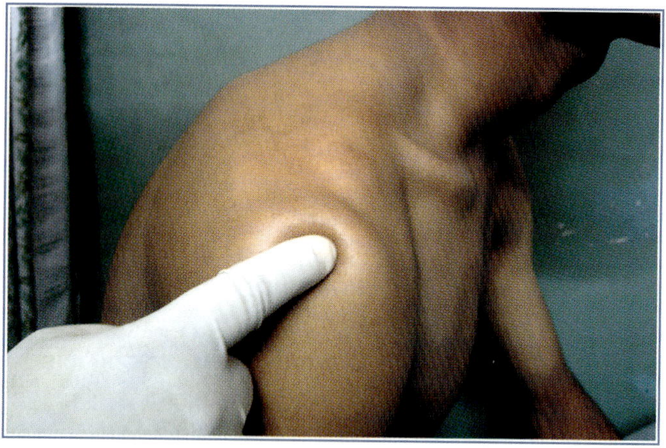

Fig. 2.11A: Identify the midpoint of the lateral edge of the acromion

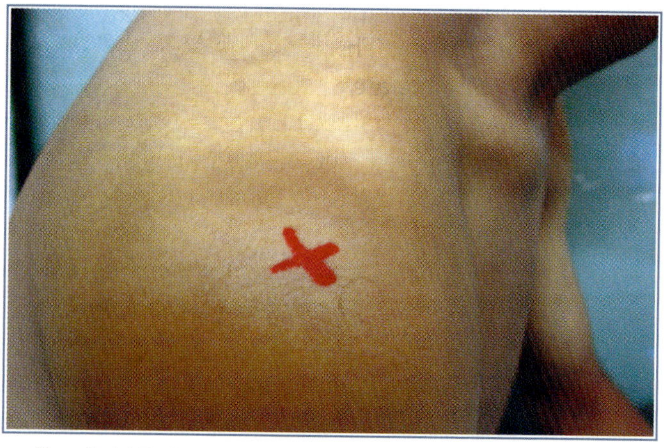

Fig. 2.11B: Mark a point just below this landmark with a sterile marker

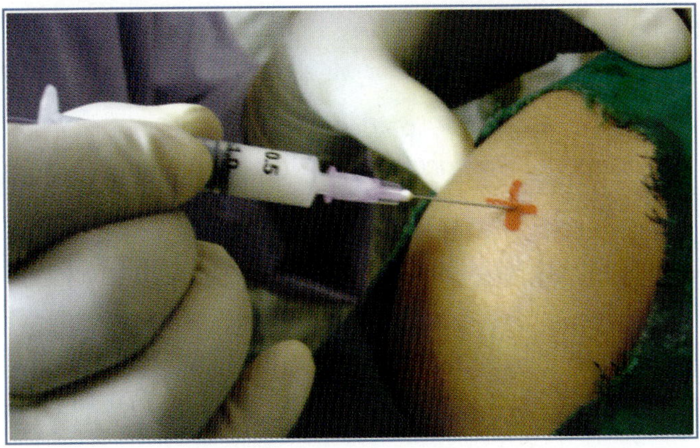

Fig. 2.11C: Advance the needle beneath the acromion process directed towards the opposite nipple

- If significant resistance is felt, the needle could be in the ligament or tendon. Withdraw or advance slightly and re-inject
- If some resistance is felt, congratulations, you are in the right space as the joint is small and the capsule is dense.

After Care

At the injection site, after the injection

- Apply ice packs
- Apply a firm sterile bandage under pressure.

Complications

- Infection (hence follow strict aseptic measures)
- Transient increase of pain (seen in 25 per cent of the cases)

- Ecchymosis
- Haematoma formation.

Note: The incidence of ecchymosis and haematoma formation can be reduced if immediately after the injection, a firm sterile pressure bandage is applied.

Vital facts: Strictly observe the following after the injection:
- Simple analgesics and NSAIDs are advised
- To prevent the exacerbation of pain, avoid heat and gentle range of motion exercises for few days
- *Avoid vigorous exercises for few days to prevent increase in pain*

AFTER CARE: At the injection site, after the injection
- Apply icepacks
- Apply a firm sterile bandage under pressure.

Frozen Shoulder

Aetiology

- Age over 40 years
- It is due to progressive adhesive capsulitis secondary to chronic inflammation of the structures of the shoulder
- More common in diabetics and collagen vascular diseases
- May be seen in patients of myocardial infarction and stroke
- Seen in fractures around the shoulder
- Women more commonly affected.

Presentation

Signs

- Difficulty in reaching behind the back as in fastening a bra

- Apley's scratch test: Here patient is unable to scratch the lower back with the affected extremity
- Inability to elevate the shoulder
- Pain is continuous and is localized to the anterolateral aspect of the shoulder. It may radiate into the lateral neck and upper anterior chest
- Grating or popping sensation may be felt
- Both active and passive range of movements are reduced.

Symptoms

- Pain around the shoulder
- Pain interteres with sleep
- Unable to lie on the affected shoulder
- Pain radiates to the outer aspect of the arm
- Patient complains of loss of shoulder range of motion.

Note: In bursitis and tendinitis only active range of movements are affected.

Late Features

- Muscle wasting
- Frozen shoulder.

Investigations

- Laboratory tests: CBC, ESR, ANA, etc
- Plain X-ray of the shoulder
- MRI if ligament rupture is suspected.

Procedures

- Position: Supine
- Preparation: Paint the shoulder with antiseptic solution
- Drape the area.

Injection Preparation

- Drugs: 0.25 per cent preservative free bupivacaine and 40 mg of methylprednisolone
- Quantity: 0.5 ml to 1 ml (due to limited capacity of the joint)
- Syringe: 2 ml/1 ½" with 25-gauge needle.

Techniques

- Locate the midpoint of the acromion
- Next identify the shoulder joint which is about one inch below the midpoint and mark it with a sterile pencil
- Paint and drape the area
- Re-identify the point marked above with a gloved finger
- Advance the needle straight at this point in this direction
- If you hit the bone, gently withdraw the needle slightly, redirect it more medially and superiorly and inject the drug.

Resistance vs Inference

- If no resistance is felt, needle could be in the joint space or the tendon could be ruptured
- If significant resistance is felt, the needle could be in the ligament or tendon. Withdraw or advance slightly and re-inject

- If some resistance is felt, congratulations, you are in the right space as the joint is small and the capsule is dense.

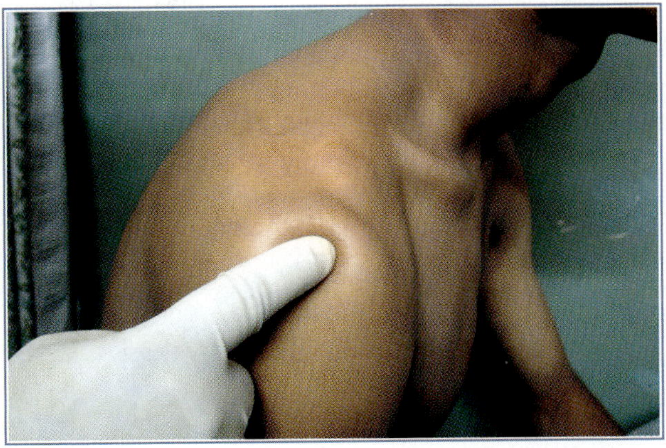

Fig. 2.12A: Identify the midpoint of the lateral edge of the acromion

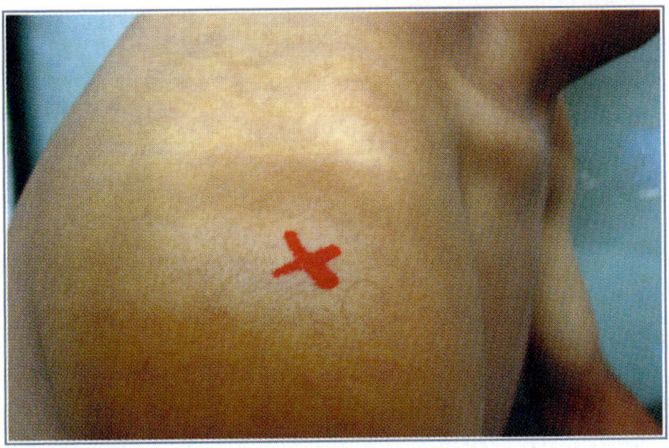

Fig. 2.12B: Mark a point just below this landmark with a sterile marker

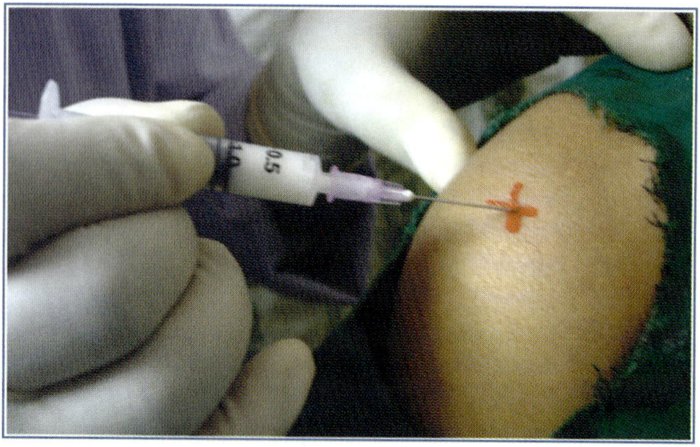

Fig. 2.12C: Advance the needle beneath the acromion process directed straight

After Care

At the injection site, after the injection

- Apply icepacks
- Apply a firm sterile bandage under pressure.

Complications

- Infection (hence follow strict aseptic measures)
- Transient increase of pain (seen in 25% of the cases)
- Ecchymosis
- Haematoma formation.

Note: The incidence of ecchymosis and haematoma formation can be reduced if immediately after the injection, a firm sterile pressure bandage is applied.

Vital facts: Strictly observe the following after the injection:
- Simple analgesics and NSAIDs are advised
- To prevent the exacerbation of pain, avoid heat and gentle range of motion exercises for few days
- Avoid vigorous exercises for few days to prevent increase in pain.

Subdeltoid Bursitis Pain

Aetiology

- Acute injuries due to direct fall
- Repetitive strain due to throwing injuries, bowling, carrying a heavy suitcases, etc.

Presentation

- Pain is brought about by any movement of the shoulder especially abduction. It is localized to the subdeltoid area. It could be referred to the insertion of the deltoid at the deltoid tuberosity on the upper one-third of the humerus
- Inability to sleep on the affected side
- On early morning awakening there is a sharp catching sensation when abducting the shoulder
- There is a point tenderness over the acromion
- There could be swelling over the deltoid
- Passive elevation and internal rotation of the affected shoulder reproduces the pain and so does resisted abduction and lateral rotation. Sudden release of resistance during this manoeuvre decreases the pain.

Investigations

- Laboratory tests: CBC, ESR, ANA, etc
- Plain X-ray of the shoulder
- MRI if ligament rupture is suspected.

Procedures

- Position: Supine
- Preparation: Paint the shoulder with antiseptic solution
- Drape the area.

Injection Preparation

- Drugs: 0.25 per cent preservative free bupivacaine and 40 mg of methylprednisolone
- Quantity: 0.5 ml to 1 ml (due to limited capacity of the joint)
- Syringe: 2 ml/1 ½" with 25-gauge needle.

Techniques

- Locate the midpoint of the acromion
- Next identify the shoulder joint which is about one inch below the midpoint and mark it with a sterile pencil
- Paint and drape the area
- Reidentify the point marked above with a gloved finger
- Advance the needle straight at this point in this direction
- If you hit the bone, gently withdraw the needle slightly, redirect it more medially and superiorly and inject the drug.

Resistance vs Inference

- If no resistance is felt, needle could be in the joint space or the tendon could be ruptured
- If significant resistance is felt, the needle could be in the ligament or tendon. Withdraw or advance slightly and re-inject
- If some resistance is felt, congratulations, you are in the right space as the joint is small and the capsule is dense.

After Care

At the injection site, after the injection

- Apply icepacks
- Apply a firm sterile bandage under pressure.

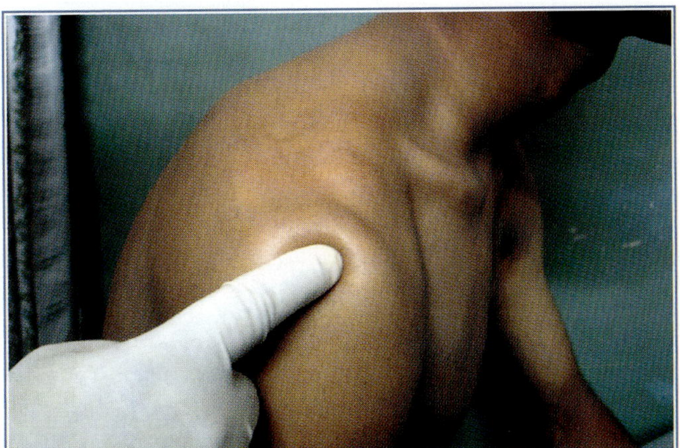

Fig. 2.13A: Identify the midpoint of the lateral edge of the acromion

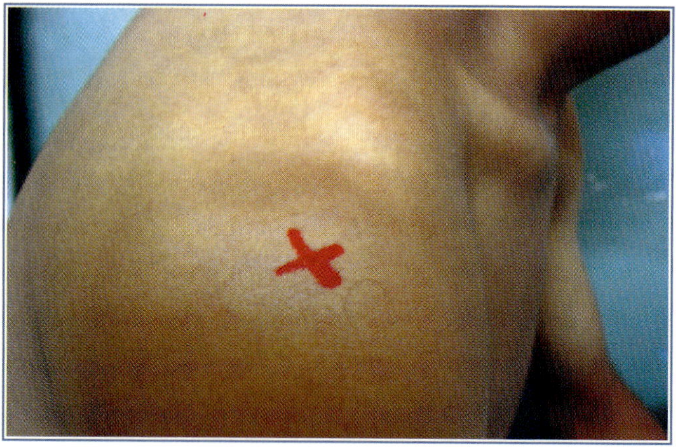

Fig. 2.13B: Mark a point just below the above of the landmark with a sterile marker

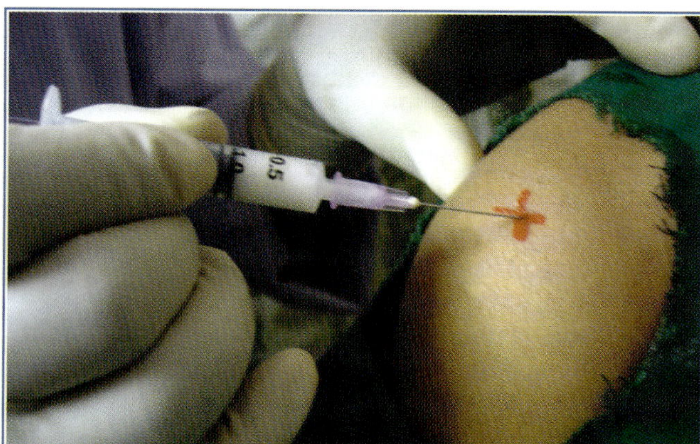

Fig. 2.13C: Advance the needle straight beneath the acromion process

Complications

- Infection (hence follow strict aseptic measures)
- Transient increase of pain (seen in 25% of the cases)
- Ecchymosis
- Haematoma formation.

Note: The incidence of ecchymosis and haematoma formation can be reduced if immediately after the injection, a firm sterile pressure bandage is applied.

Vital facts: Strictly observe the following after the injection:
- Simple analgesics and NSAIDs are advised
- To prevent the exacerbation of pain, avoid heat and gentle range of motion exercises for few days
- Avoid vigorous exercises for few days to prevent increase in pain.

Subcoracoid Bursitis

Aetiology

- Direct trauma to the shoulder
- Due to repeated strain.

Presentation

- Pain is localized over the coracoid process with referred pain noted at the medial shoulder
- Point tenderness over the coracoid process
- Inability to sleep on the affected side
- Passive elevation and medial rotation of the affected shoulder reproduces the pain

- Resisted adduction and medial rotation and sudden release of resistance markedly increases the pain.

Investigations

- Laboratory tests: CBC, ESR, ANA, etc
- Plain X-ray of the shoulder
- MRI if ligament rupture is suspected.

Procedures

- Position: Supine
- Preparation: Paint the shoulder with antiseptic solution. Drape the area.

Injection Preparation

- Drugs: 0.25 per cent preservative free bupivacaine and 40 mg of methylprednisolone
- Quantity: 4 ml
- Syringe: 2 ml/1 ½ " with 25-gauge needle.

Techniques

- In the above position, identify the anterior surface of the lateral end of the clavicle
- Next identify the deepest portion of the clavicle concavity
- One inch below this point the coracoid process can be felt by deep palpation
- Mark it with a sterile pencil
- Paint and drape the area
- Re-identify the point marked above with a gloved finger

- Advance the needle through the skin in a posterior and lateral direction, just beneath the coracoid process
- If you hit the bone, gently withdraw the needle slightly, redirect it more inferiorly and inject the drug.

Resistance vs Inference

- If significant resistance is felt, the needle could be in the ligament or tendon. Withdraw or advance slightly and re-inject
- If minimal resistance is felt, congratulations, you are in the right spot.

After Care

At the injection site, after the injection

- Apply icepacks
- Apply a firm sterile bandage under pressure.

Complications

- Infection (hence follow strict aseptic measures)
- Transient increase of pain (seen in 25% of the cases)
- Ecchymosis
- Haematoma formation.

Note: The incidence of ecchymosis and haematoma formation can be reduced if immediately after the injection, a firm sterile pressure bandage is applied.

Vital facts: Strictly observe the following after the injection:

- Simple analgesics and NSAIDs are advised
- To prevent the exacerbation of pain, avoid heat and gentle range of motion exercises for few days
- Avoid vigorous exercises for few days to prevent increase in pain.

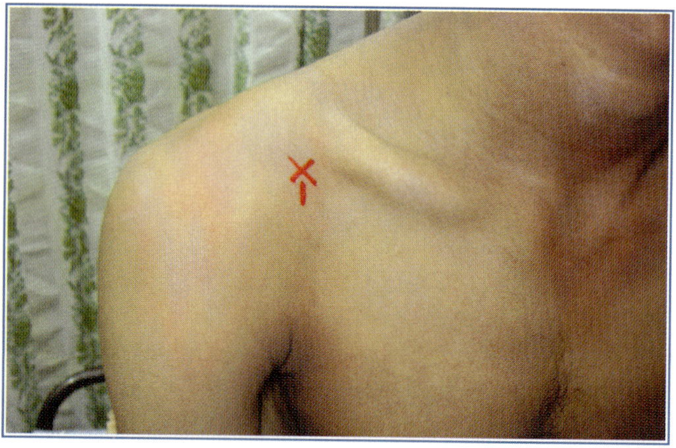

Fig. 2.14A: Identify the anterior surface of the concavity of the lateral end of the clavicle. Mark a point one inch below this that overlies the coracoid process

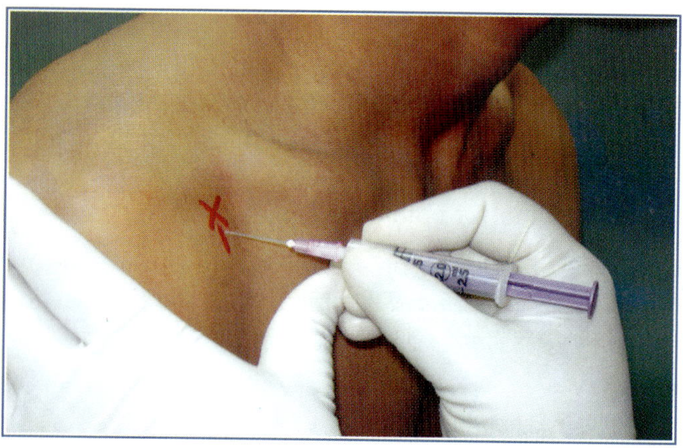

Fig. 2.14B: Advance the needle in a posterior and lateral direction just beneath the coracoid process

ELBOW COMPLEX

INJECTION IN AND AROUND THE ELBOW

Intra-articular Injections into the Elbow Joint

The approaches commonly employed are the anterolateral approach and the posterior approach.

a. *The anterolateral approach (towards the humeroradial joint line):* This consists of the following steps:
   - The elbow is kept flexed at 90 degrees and is resting on a firm surface
   - Palpate the head of the radius while passively supinating and pronating the patient's forearm
   - This enables to identify the joint line
   - Insert the needle tangentially towards the joint line from a superolateral angle
   - Aim to place the needle tip just beneath the capsule and deep between the two bones.

b. Posterior approach (towards the olecranon fossa)
   - Patient is in the same position mentioned above
   - Palpate the olecranon process,the para-olecranon grooves and the olecranon fossa
   - Insert the needle into the olecranon fossa just above and lateral to the superior aspect of the olecranon.

Aetiology

- Osteoarthritis of the elbow is the most common cause of arthritis
- Rheumatoid arthritis

- Post-traumatic arthritis
- Psoriatic arthritis
- Diagnosis of radial head fracture (Blood or fat globules in aspiration).

Less Common Cause

- Collagen vascular disease
- Infection
- Lyme's disease.

Presentation

- Pain around the elbow and forearm
- Rest relieves the pain and activity worsens it
- Pain is constant and interferes with sleep
- Patient may complain of grating or popping sensation
- Crepitus could be felt.

Late

- Decrease in functional ability with decreased range of movements
- Muscle wasting
- Ankylosis.

Investigation

- Laboratory tests: CBC, ESR, ANA test, etc.
- Plain X-ray of the elbow
- MRI if joint instability is suspected.

Procedures

- Position: Supine with the arm fully adducted at the patients side and the elbow flexed at 45° with the dorsum of the hand resting on a small pillow
- Drugs: 5 ml of local anaesthetics and 40 mg of methylprednisolone
- Syringe: 12 ml/1 " length/25-gauge.

Techniques

- Put the patient in the position mentioned above
- At the posterolateral aspect of the elbow identify the head of the radius
- Identify the indentation between the radial head and the humerus. Mark this poit with a sterile marker
- Paint and drape the area
- Re-identify the marked point with a gloved finger
- Advanced the needle through the skin and subcutaneous tissue along the point marked
- If you hit the bone, withdraw and redirect the needle more superiorly
- After entering the joint space gently inject the drugs.

Reisitance vs Inference

- If significant resistance is felt, the needle could be in the ligament or tendon. Withdraw or advance slightly and re-inject
- If minimal resistance is felt, congratulations, you are in the right space and within the joint.

After Care

At the injection site, after the injection

- Apply icepacks
- Apply a firm sterile bandage under pressure.

Complications

- Infection (hence follow strict aseptic measures)
- Transient increase of pain (seen in 25% of the cases)
- Ecchymosis
- Haematoma formation.

Note: The incidence of ecchymosis and haematoma formation can be reduced if immediately after the injection, a firm sterile pressure bandage is applied.

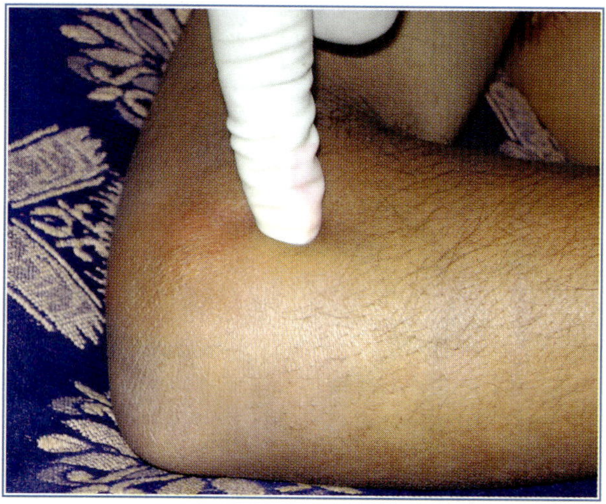

Fig. 2.15A: Identify the lateral epicondyle

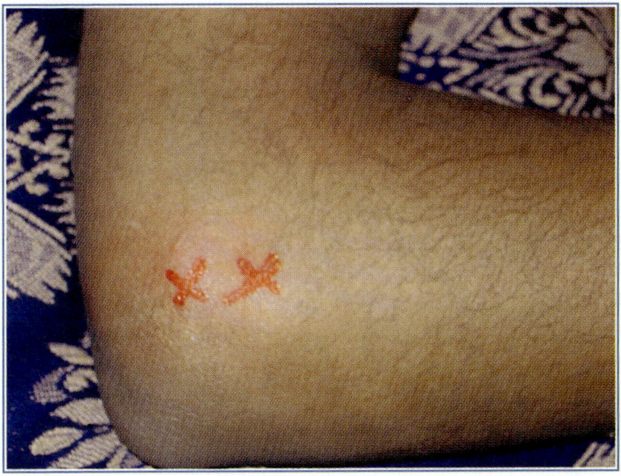

Fig. 2.15B: Identify the indentation beneath the lateral epicondyle and mark it. This represents the radial head

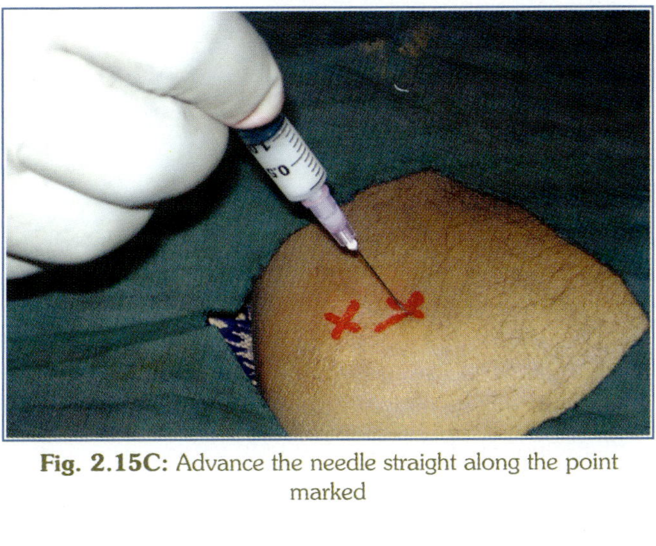

Fig. 2.15C: Advance the needle straight along the point marked

Vital facts: Strictly observe the following after the injection:
- Simple analgesics and NSAID'S are advised
- To prevent the exacerbation of pain, avoid heat and gentle range of motion exercises for few days
- Avoid vigorous exercises for few days to prevent increase in pain

LOCAL INFILTRATION OF INJECTION FOR SOFT TISSUE LESIONS AROUND THE ELBOW

Tennis Elbow

Causes: It is due to repetitive microtrauma to the common extensor tendons of the forearm; namely the extensor carpi radialis brevis and extensor carpi ulnaris. The acute inflammation may become chronic due to repeated overuse or misuse of these forearm extensors.

Who is Vulnerable?

It is more common in people who are involved in repetitive activities that involve hand grasping:
- Politicians shaking the hands
- People involved in scooping ice-cream at an ice-cream parlor
- Tennis players: Due to increased pressure grip strain resulting from the use of heavy racquet or backhand strokes with leading shoulder and elbow rather than keeping them parallel to the net.

Presentation

- Pain is localized to the lateral epicondyle
- Pain is constant and it increases with active contraction of the wrist
- Patient complains of inability to hold a coffee cup or hammer
- Sleep disturbance is common
- Elbow range of movements is normal
- Grip strength on the affected side is reduced
- Positive Tennis elbow test (Cozen's test)
- The tenderness in tennis elbow is maximum on the lateral epicondyle whereas in radial tunnel syndrome it is just distal to the lateral epicondyle.

Investigation

- Laboratory tests: CBC, ESR, ANA test, etc.
- Plain X-ray of the elbow
- MRI if joint instability is suspected
- Injection technique: It is both diagnostic and therapeutic.

Procedures

- Position: Supine or sitting with the arm fully adducted at the patient's side and the elbow flexed to 45° with the dorsum of the hand resting on a small pillow or folded towel to relax the affected tendons in pronation
- Drugs: 5 ml of local anaesthetics and 40 mg of methylprednisolone
- Syringe: 5 ml/1 " length/25-gauge.

Techniques

- In the position mentioned above identify the lateral epicondyle and mark it with a sterile marker
- Paint and drape the area
- Re-identify the point of '*maximum tenderness*' with a gloved finger
- Advance the needle perpendicular to the lateral epicondyle through the skin till it touches the bone
- Now slightly withdraw the needle by 1 to 2 mm and inject both deeply (i.e as near to the bone as possible) and also superficially by a fan technique of half withdrawals and reinsertions
- Here the injection is made under pressure.

Reisitance vs Inference

- If significant resistance is felt, the needle could be in the ligament or tendon. Withdraw or advance slightly and re-inject
- If minimal resistance is felt, congratulations, you are in the right space and within the joint.

After Care

At the injection site, after the injection

- Apply icepacks
- Apply a firm sterile bandage under pressure.

Complications

- Infection (hence follow strict aseptic measures)
- Transient increase of pain (seen in 25% of the cases)

- Ecchymosis
- Haematoma formation
- Neakening of tendon insertion.

Note: The incidence of ecchymosis and haematoma formation can be reduced if immediately after the injection, a firm sterile pressure bandage is applied.

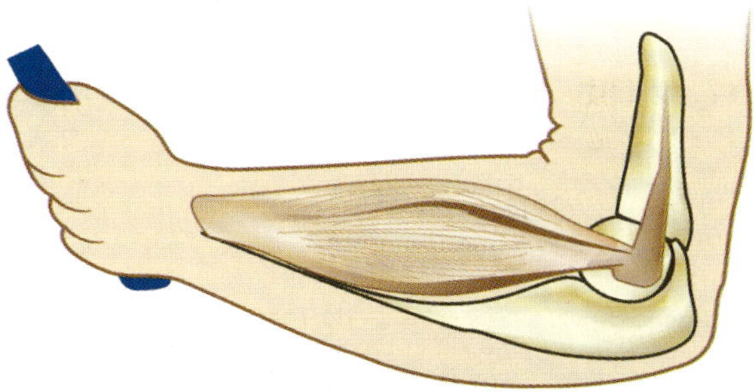

Fig. 2.16A: Showing the point of origin of common extensor group of muscles

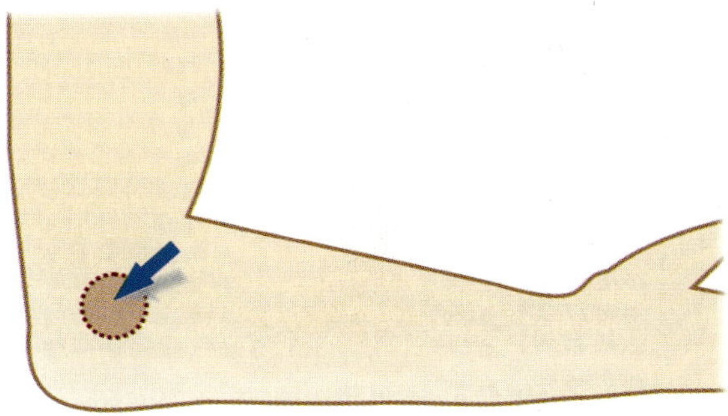

Fig. 2.16B: Showing the point of tenderness in tennis elbow

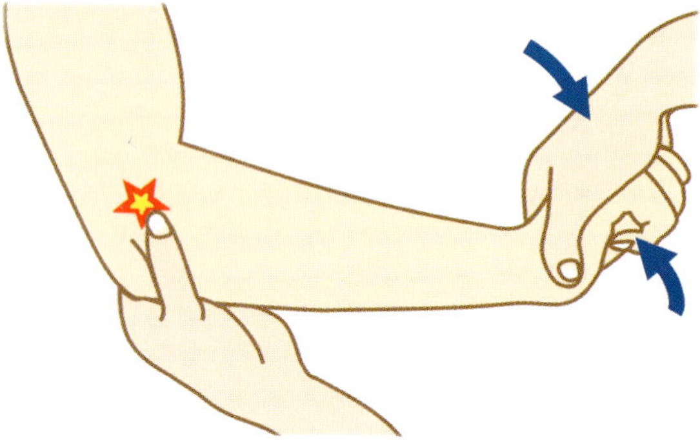

Fig. 2.16C: Showing the method of performing the Cozen's test

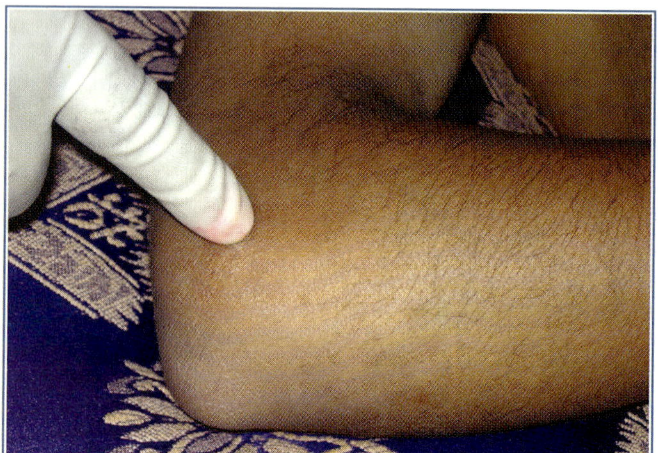

Fig. 2.16D: Identify the lateral epicondyle

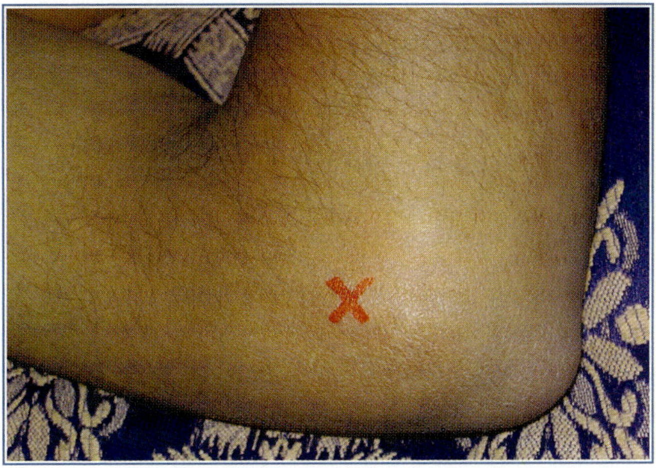

Fig. 2.16E: Mark it with a sterile marker

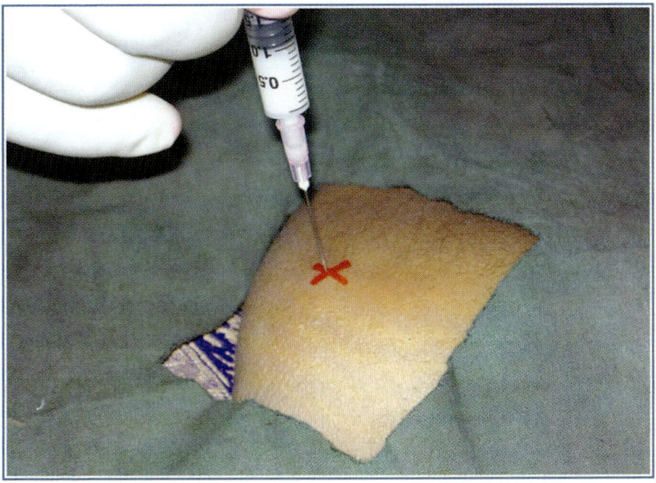

Fig. 2.16F: Advance the needle perpendicular to the lateral epicondyle

Vital facts: Strictly observe the following after the injection:
- Simple analgesics and NSAIDs are advised
- To prevent the exacerbation of pain, avoid heat and gentle range of motion exercises for few days
- Avoid vigorous exercises for few days to prevent increase in pain.

Radial Tunnel Syndrome

Definition: It is an entrapment neuropathy involving the posterior interosseous branch of the radial nerve.

Mechanism: The entrapment could be due to:
- Aberrant fibrous bands in front of the radial nerve
- Anomalous blood vessels compressing the nerve
- Sharp tendinous margin of the extensor carpi radialis brevis.

Pitfall: It is often confused and mistaken for tennis elbow.

Presentation

- Pain just below the lateral epicondyle
- It starts after an acute twisting injury or after direct trauma to the soft tissues. In some cases the onset could be insidious.
- If pain is constant and is made worse with active supination of the wrist
- Patient could complain of inability to hold coffee cup or hammer
- Sleep disturbance is common
- Tenderness to palpation just below the lateral epicondyle
- Elbow range of movements is normal

- Grip strength on the affected side is weak
- Patient exhibits pain on active resisted supination of the forearm.

Differencial Diagnosis

- Tennis elbow: Maximal tenderness is on the lateral epicondyle
- Cervical radiculopathy is identified by ENG studies.

Investigation

- Laboratory tests: CBC, ESR, ANA test, etc.
- Plain X-ray of the elbow: To rule out occult bony pathology
- MRI if joint instability is suspected
- Injection technique: It is both diagnostic and therapeutic.

Procedures

- Position: Supine or sitting with the arm adducted by 35 to 40 degrees at the patient's side and the elbow flexed with the spalm of the hand resting on the abdomen
- Drugs: local an anaesthetics and 120 mg of Methylprednisolone
- Syringe: 12 ml/1 "length/25 gauge
- A 7 to 10 ml of the mixture of local anaesthetics and 810 mg of methylprednisolone is given as the first block. The second block consists of 40 mg of methylprednisolone.

Techniques

- In the position mentioned above identify the lateral epicondyle
- About three inches above the lateral epicondyle, with deep palpation identify the musculospiral groove between the heads of the triceps muscle. Mark it with a sterile marker
- Paint and drape the area
- Re-identify the point with a gloved finger
- Advance the needle perpendicular to the lateral aspect of the humerus through the skin and advance it slowly towards the musculospiral groove
- If bone is encountered slightly withdraw the needle and re-inject
- If you hit the right spot, there will be paraesthesia along the course of the radial nerve
- If you hit the bone or if no paraesthesia is elicited, then withdraw the needle and redirect it slightly more anterior or posterior until paraesthesia is elicited
- Before injecting the drugs, gently aspirate. If the aspiration test is negative, and if there is no persistent paraesthesia, inject about 7 to 20 ml of the solution.

After Care

At the injection site, after the injection

- Apply icepacks
- Apply a firm sterile bandage under pressure.

Complications

- Infection (hence follow strict aseptic measures)
- Transient increase of pain (seen in 25% of the cases)
- Ecchymosis
- Haematoma formation.

Note: The incidence of ecchymosis and haematoma formation can be reduced if immediately after the injection, a firm sterile pressure bandage is applied.

Vital facts: Strictly observe the following after the injection:
- Simple analgesics and NSAIDs are advised
- To prevent the exacerbation of pain, avoid heat and gentle range of motion exercises for few days
- Avoid vigorous exercises for few days to prevent increase in pain.

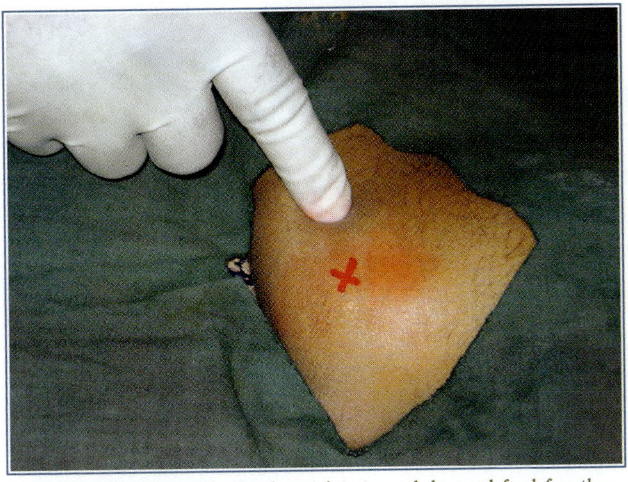

Fig.2.17A: Identify the lateral epicondyle and feel for the lateral supracondylar ridge above this point

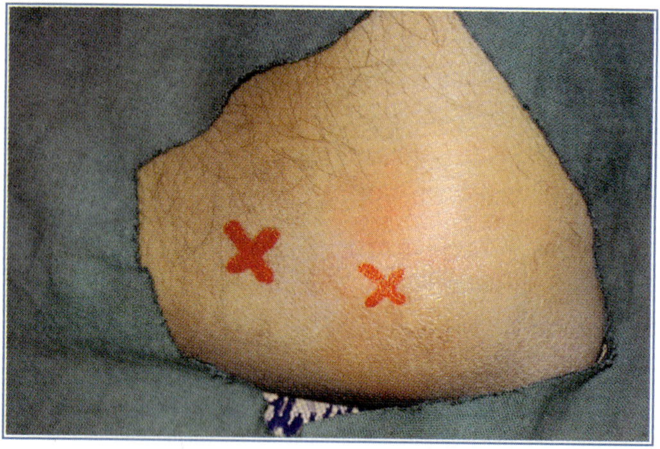

Fig. 2.17B: Mark a point about three inches above the lateral epicondyle with a sterile marker

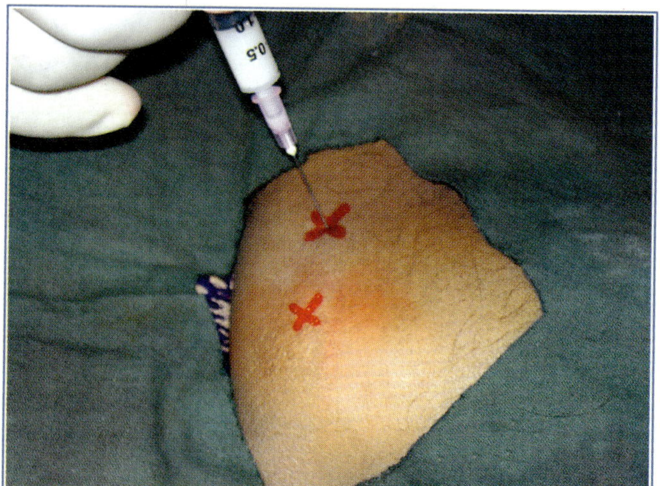

Fig. 2.17C: Advance the needle perpendicular to the lateral aspect of the humerus

Golfer's Elbow

Definition: It is due to repetitive microtrauma to the flexor tendons of the forearm or at their origins; namely the pronator teres, flexor carpi radialis, and flexor carpi ulnaris and palamaris longus.

Who is Vulnerable?

People engaged in repetitive flexion activities like:

- Baseball players
- Carrying heavy suitcases
- Golfball players.

Presentation

- Pain localized to the medial epicondyle
- Pain is constant and is made worse by active contraction of the wrist
- Patient complains of inability to hold a coffee cup or hammer
- Sleep disturbance is common.

Findings

- Tenderness on or just below the medial epicondyle
- Elbow range of movements is normal
- Grip strength is decreased
- *Golfer's* elbow test: patient complains of pain on attempting to flex the wrist against resistance.

Investigations

- Laboratory tests: CBC, ESR, ANA test, etc.
- Plain X-ray of the elbow
- MRI if joint instability is suspected
- Injection technique: It is both diagnostic and therapeutic.

Procedures

- Position: Supine or sitting with the arm abducted at the patient's side and the elbow fully extended or flexed 45° with the dorsum of the hand (supination) resting on a small pillow or folded towel to relax the affected tendons
- Drugs: 1 ml of local anaesthetics and 40 mg of methylprednisolone
- Syringe: 5 ml/1 " length/25-gauge.

Techniques

- In the position mentioned above identify the medial epicondyle and mark it with a sterile marker at the most tender spot
- Paint and drape the area
- Re-identify the point with a gloved finger
- Advance the needle perpendicular to the medial epicondyle through the skin
- If bone is encountered slightly withdraw the needle and re-inject.

Reisitance vs Inference

- If significant resistance is felt, the needle could be in the ligament or tendon. Withdraw or advance slightly and re-inject
- If minimal resistance is felt, congratulations, you are in the right space and within the joint.

After Care

At the injection site, after the injection
- Apply ice packs
- Apply a firm sterile bandage under pressure.

Complications

- Infection (hence follow strict aseptic measures)
- Transient increase of pain (seen in 25% of the cases)
- Ecchymosis
- Haematoma formation
- Injury to ulnar nerve.

Note: The incidence of ecchymosis and haematoma formation can be reduced if immediately after the injection, a firm sterile pressure bandage is applied.

Vital facts: Strictly observe the following after the injection:
- Simple analgesics and NSAIDs are advised
- To prevent the exacerbation of pain, avoid heat and gentle range of motion exercises for few days
- Avoid vigorous exercises for few days to prevent increase in pain.

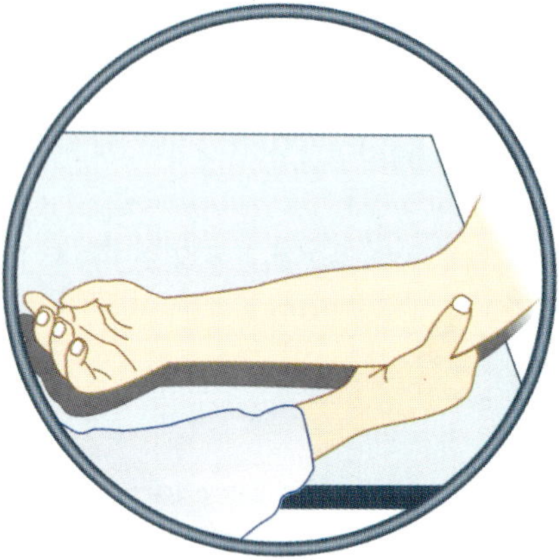

Fig. 2.18A: Method of eliciting tenderness in golfer's elbow

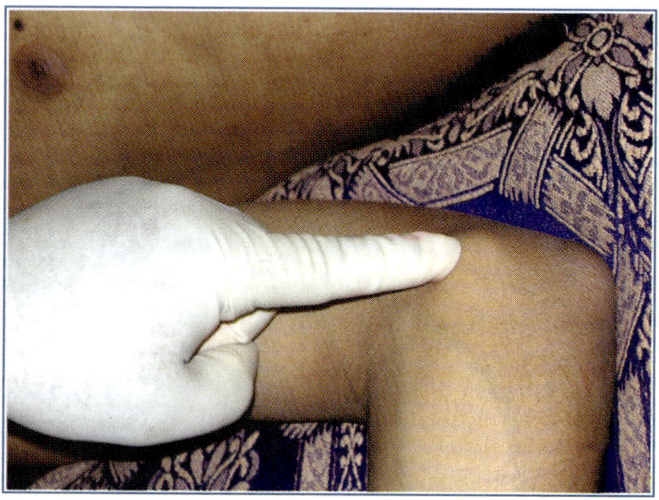

Fig. 2.18B: Identify the medial epicondyle

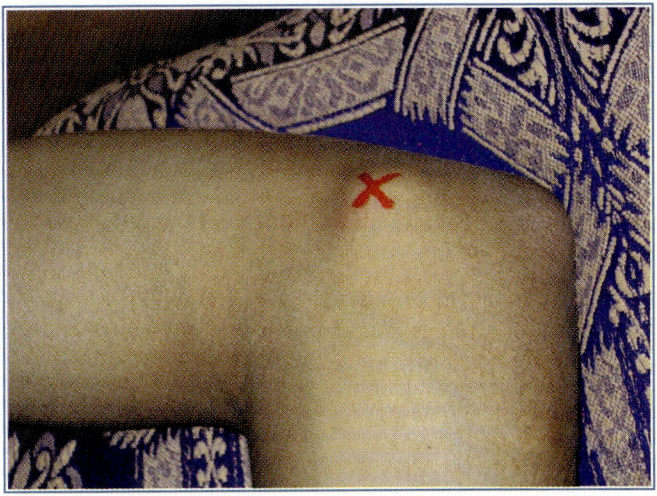

Fig. 2.18C: Mark it with a sterile marker

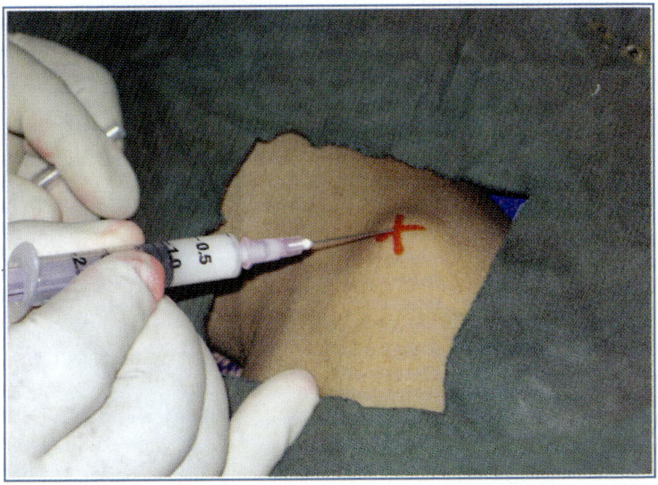

Fig. 2.18D: Advance the needle perpendicular to the medial epicondyle

Student's Elbow (Olecranon Bursitis Pain)

Olecranon bursa lies between the olecranon process and the skin.

Causes

- Direct trauma to the back of the elbow due to fall, assault, sports, etc
- More commonly it is due to chronic repetitive friction due to the habit of leaning over the elbow over a desk or table while working, reading, etc.

Other Causes

- Gout
- Infection.

Presentation

- Pain often referred above the elbow
- Swelling is a more important complaint than the pain.

Note: Though pain and swelling can be seen in any movement of the elbow, it is more commonly seen in extension.

- Pain increases on direct pressure or on passive extension and resisted shoulder flexion
- In infected bursa patient may present with fever and chills.

Investigation

- Laboratory tests: CBC, ESR, ANA test, etc. Gram stain and culture if infection is suspected
- Plain X-ray of the elbow.

Procedures

- Position: Supine or sitting with the arm fully adducted at the patient's side and the elbow flexed with the dorsum of the hand resting on a small pillow or folded towel or on the patients abdomen to relax the affected tendons
- Drugs: 2 ml of local anaesthetics and 40 mg of methylprednisolone
- Syringe: 5 ml/1 " length/25-gauge.

Techniques

- In the position mentioned above identify the olecranon process and mark it with a sterile marker
- Paint and drape the area
- Re-identify the point with a gloved finger
- Advance the needle directly into the middle of the bursa through the skin
- If bone is encountered slightly withdraw the needle and re-inject the contents of the syringe slowly
- Remove the needle, apply icepacks and pressure bandages.

Resistance vs Inference

- If significant resistance is felt, the needle could be in the ligament or tendon. Withdraw or advance slightly and re-inject
- If minimal resistance is felt, congratulations, you are in the right space and within the joint.

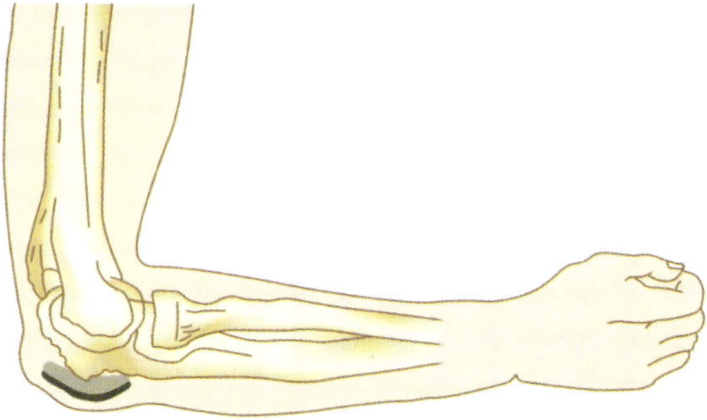

Fig. 2.19A: Showing the presence of olecranon bursa

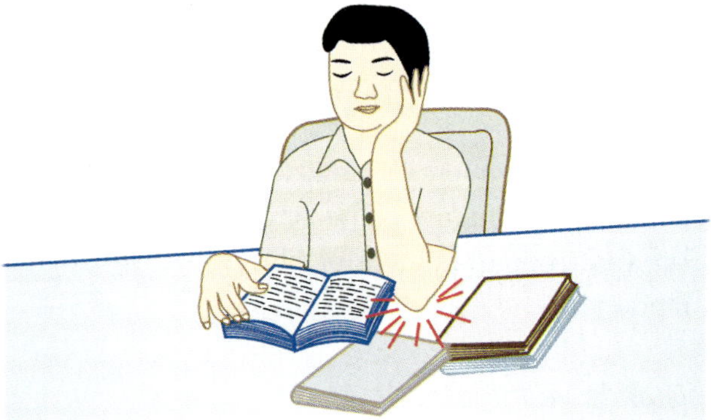

Fig. 2.19B: Mechanism of the formation of olecranon bursitis

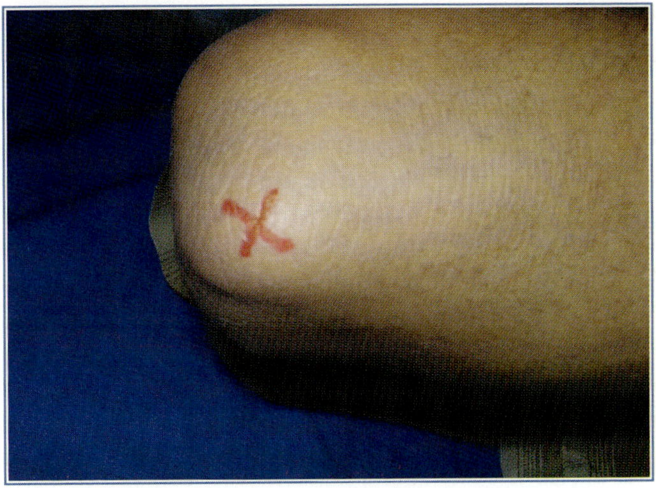

Fig. 2.19C: Mark the centre of the olecranon bursa with a sterile marker

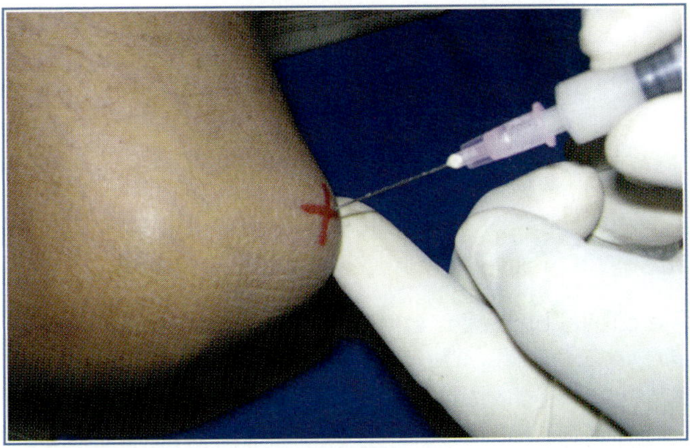

Fig. 2.19D: Insert the needle perpendicular to the marked point and inject

After Care

At the injection site, after the injection

- Apply icepacks
- Apply a firm sterile bandage under pressure.

Complications

- Infection (hence follow strict aseptic measures)
- Transient increase of pain (seen in 25% of the cases)
- Injury to the ulnar nerve
- Ecchymosis
- Haematoma formation.

Note: The incidence of ecchymosis and haematoma formation can be reduced if immediately after the injection, a firm sterile pressure bandage is applied.

Vital facts: Strictly observe the following after the injection:

- Simple analgesics and NSAIDs are advised
- To prevent the exacerbation of pain, avoid heat and gentle range of motion exercises for few days
- Avoid vigorous exercises for few days to prevent increase in pain.

Cubital Bursitis

The cubital bursa lies in the anterior aspect of the elbow.

Aetiology

- Acute injuries due to direct trauma to the exterior aspect of the elbow

- Due to repetitive micro trauma to the elbow as in javelin and baseball sportsperson
- Gout or rheumatoid arthritis.

Presentation

- Pain and swelling with any movement of the elbow
- Pain is mainly localized to the cubital area but may radiate to the forearm and hand
- Point tenderness in the anterior aspect of the elbow
- Swelling due to bursa in the cubital fossa
- Pain is reproduced by direct pressure and by passive extension and resisted elbow flexion.

Investigations

- Laboratory tests: CBC, ESR, ANA test, etc.
- Plain X-ray of the elbow may reveal calcification of the bursa if present.

Procedures

- Position: Supine or sitting with the arm fully adducted at the patient's side and the elbow extended with the dorsum of the hand resting on a small pillow or folded towel to relax the affected tandons
- Drugs: 2 ml of local anaesthetics and 40 mg of methylprednisolone
- Syringe: 5 ml/1 " length/25-gauge.

Techniques

- In the position mentioned above feel for the pulsations of the brachial artery at the elbow and mark it with a sterile marker
- Paint and drape the area
- Re-identify the point with a gloved finger
- Advance the needle just lateral to the artery in a slightly medial and cephalad direction through the skin
- If bone is encountered slightly withdraw the needle and re-inject.

Resistance vs Inference

- If significant resistance is felt, the needle could be in the ligament or tendon. Withdraw or advance slightly and re-inject
- If minimal resistance is felt; congratulations, you are in the right space and within the joint.

After Care

At the injection site, after the injection

- Apply icepacks
- Apply a firm sterile bandage under pressure.

Complications

- Infection (hence follow strict aseptic measures)
- Transient increase of pain (seen in 25% of the cases)
- Ecchymosis
- Haematoma formation.

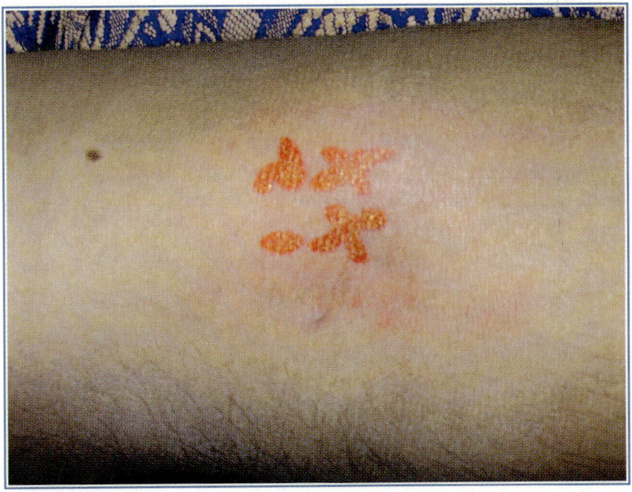

Fig. 2.20A: Feel for the pulsations of the brachial artery lateral to the medial epicondyle and mark it

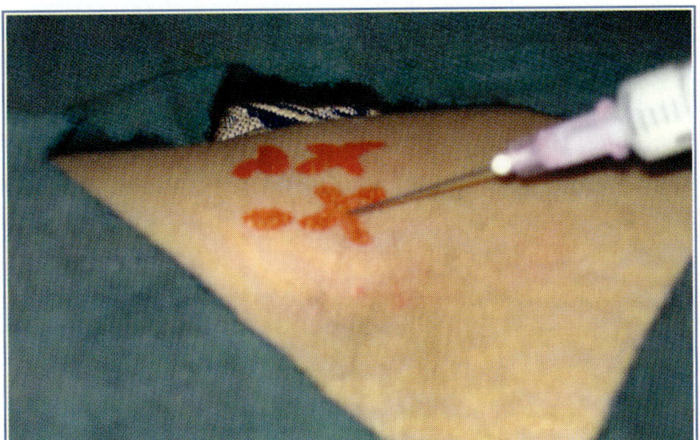

Fig. 2.20B: Just lateral to the brachial artery mark another point. Advance the needle through this point in a slightly cephalad and medial direction

Note: The incidence of ecchymosis and haematoma formation can be reduced if immediately after the injection, a firm sterile pressure bandage is applied.

Vital facts: Strictly observe the following after the injection:
- Simple analgesics and NSAIDs are advised
- To prevent the exacerbation of pain, avoid heat and gentle range of motion exercises for few days
- Avoid vigorous exercises for few days to prevent increase in pain.

Cubital Tunnel Syndrome

This is an entrapment neuropathy of the ulnar nerve by an aponeurotic band that runs from the medial epicondyle of the humerus to the medial border of the humerus.

Presentation

- Presents as pain and paraesthesiae in the lateral forearm that radiate to the wrist, ring and little fingers
- Late stages there could be flexion contracture of the affected finger
- Tenderness is present over the ulnar nerve at the elbow in the early stages
- Tinel's sign is positive
- Loss of sensation over the one and half fingers is also early a sign.

Causes

- Repeated elbow movements
- Repeated pressure on the elbow (as in using elbow to rise from the bed)
- Direct injury to the ulnar nerve.

Importance

It is often confused with Golfer's elbow and fails to respond to conservative treatment. In Golfer's elbow tenderness is over the medial epicondyle while in the cubital tunnel syndrome tenderness is one inch below the medial epicondyle.

Investigation

- Laboratory tests: CBC, ESR, ANA test, etc.
- Plain X-ray of the elbow
- MRI if joint instability is suspected
- Injection technique: It is both diagnostic and therapeutic.

Procedures

- Position: Supine or sitting with the arm fully adducted at the patient's side and the elbow flexed with the dorsum of the hand resting on a small pillow or folded towel to relax the affected tendons
- Drugs: 5 ml of local anaesthetics and 40 mg of methylprednisolone
- Syringe: 12 ml/1 " length/25-gauge
- A 5 to 7 ml of local anaesthetics and 80 mg of methylprednisolone is given as the first block. Next add 40 mg of methylprednisolon as the second block.

Techniques

- In the position mentioned above identify the olecranon process and medial epicondyle

- Next identify the sulcus between them and mark it with a sterile marker
- Paint and drape the area
- Re-identify the point with a gloved finger
- Insert the needle just proximal to the sulcus and advance it in a slightly cephalad direction through the skin
- After advancing the needle for half an inch a strong paraesthesia should be elicited in the distribution of the ulnar nerve
- Once paraesthesia is felt, aspirate for the presence of blood
- If aspiration test is negative and if there is no persistent paraesthesia, inject 5 to 7 ml of the solution slowly.

Note: If no paraesthesia is encountered, then inject the drug in a fanlike manner just proximal to the notch.

- If bone is encountered slightly withdraw the needle and re-inject.

Resistance vs Inference

- If significant resistance is felt, the needle could be in the ligament or tendon. Withdraw or advance slightly and re-inject
- If minimal resistance is felt, congratulations, you are in the right space and within the joint.

After Care

At the injection site, after the injection

- Apply icepacks
- Apply a firm sterile bandage under pressure.

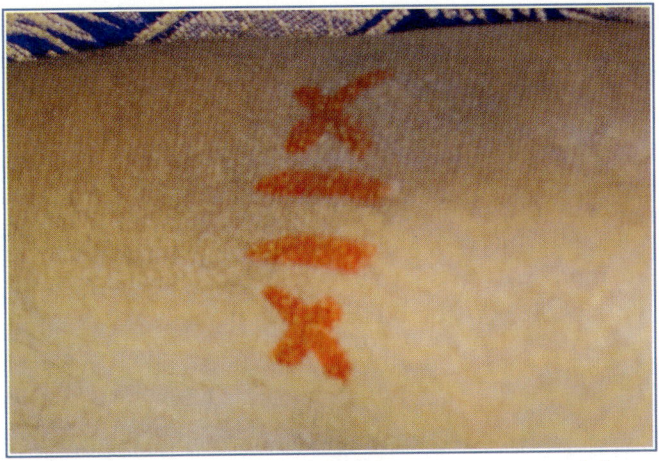

Fig. 2.21A: Feel and mark the olecranon process and the medial epicondyle

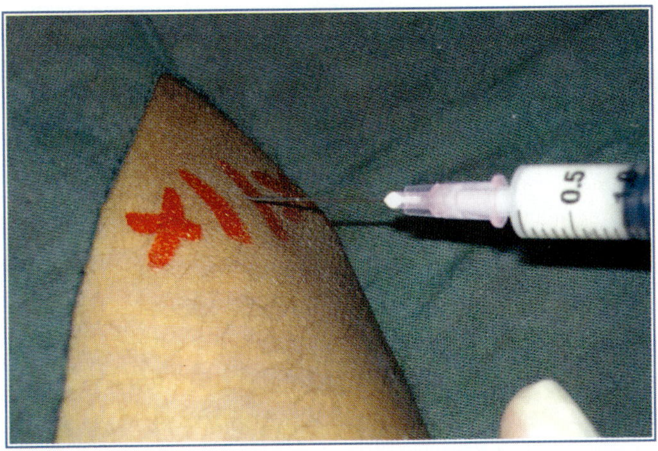

Fig. 2.21B: Feel for the sulcus between these two points. Advance the needle through this point in a slightly cephalad direction

Complications

- Infection (hence follow strict aseptic measures)
- Transient increase of pain (seen in 25% of the cases)
- Ecchymosis
- Haematoma formation.

Note: The incidence of ecchymosis and haematoma formation can be reduced if immediately after the injection, a firm sterile pressure bandage is applied.

Vital facts: Strictly observe the following after the injection:
- Simple analgesics and NSAIDs are advised
- To prevent the exacerbation of pain, avoid heat and gentle range of motion exercises for few days
- Avoid vigorous exercises for few days to prevent increase in pain.

WRIST AND HAND COMPLEX

WRIST

Intra-articular Injection into the Wrist Joint

In the wrist injection is usually done into the radiocarpal joints or just inferior the ulnar styloid process. The steps suggested are as follows:

- Identify the joint space by careful palpation
- Hold the wrist in partially flexed position
- Inject using a superior approach to the joint space just medial to the ulnar styloid process or lateral to the extensor pollicis longus tendon.

Causes

- Osteoarthritis
- Rheumatoid arthritis
- Post-traumatic arthritis
- Psoriatic arthritis.

Less Common

- Collagen vascular disease
- Infection
- Lyme's disease.

Presentation

- Wrist pain localized to wrist and hand
- Pain is continuous and aching in nature
- Pain worsens with activity and lessens with heat and rest
- The pain may interfere with sleep
- There could be a grating sensation and crepitus could be felt.

Late

- Gradual decrease in functional activity, simple everyday tasks are affected
- Muscle wasting may be seen.

Investigations

- Laboratory tests: This includes CBC, ESR, ANA tests, etc.
- Plain X-ray of the wrist
- MRI.

Procedures

- Position: Supine with arm fully adducted at the patient's side and the elbow slightly flexed with the palm of the hand resting on a small pillow
- Drugs: 1.5 ml of local anaesthetics and 40 mg of methylprednisolone
- Syringe: 5 ml/1"/25-gauge needle.

Techniques

- Paint and drape the area around the wrist
- Identify the mid carpus which lies proximal to the indentation of the capitate bone
- There is an indentation just proximal to the capitate bone which allows easy access into the wrist
- Advance the needle through this point
- If you hit the bone, withdraw and redirect the needle superiorly
- Inject the contents of the syringe into the joint space.

Resistance vs Inference

- *If there is significant resistance:* The needle could be in the ligament is tendon. Advance it slightly into the joint space
- *If there is least resistance;* congratulations you have hit the right spot.

After Care

At the injection site, after the injection

- Apply icepacks
- Apply a firm sterile bandage under pressure.

Complications

- Infection (hence follow strict aseptic measures)
- Transient increase of pain (seen in 25% of the cases)
- Ecchymosis
- Haematoma formation.

Note: The incidence of ecchymosis and haematoma formation can be reduced if immediately after the injection, a firm sterile pressure bandage is applied.

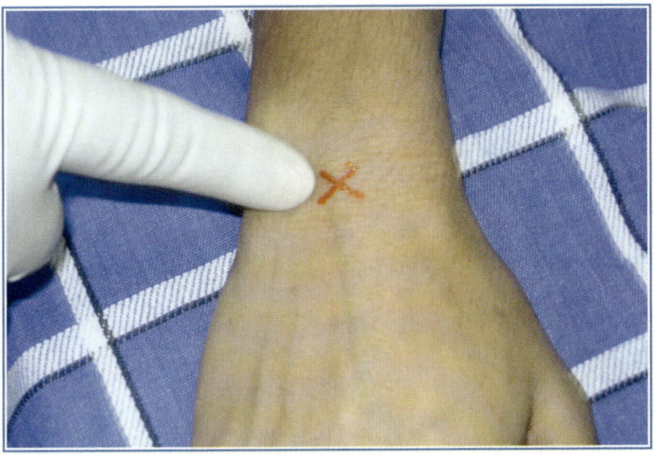

Fig. 2.22A: Identify the mipoint of the carpus

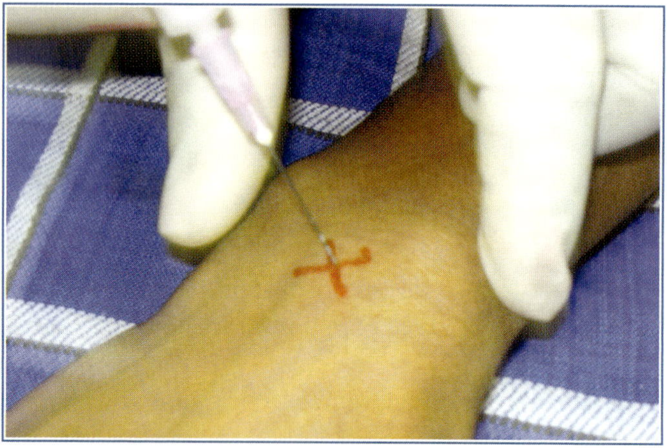

Fig. 2.22B: Advance the needle straight through this point

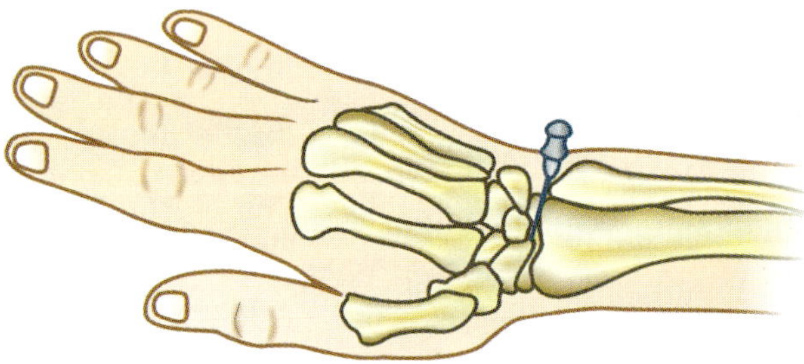

Fig. 2.22C: Needle depicted as inside the joint

Vital facts: Strictly observe the following after the injection:

- Simple analgesics and NSAIDs are advised
- To prevent the exacerbation of pain, avoid heat and gentle range of motion exercises for few days
- Avoid vigorous exercises for few days to prevent increase in pain.

The Distal Radioulnar Joint

Causes of Pain

- Osteoarthritis
- Rheumatoid arthritis
- Post-traumatic arthritis
- Psoriatic arthritis.

Rare Causes

- Collagen vascular disease
- Lyme's disease
- Infection.

Presentation

- Pain is localized to the distal forearm
- Pronation and supination activity makes the pain worse
- Pain is relieved by rest and heat
- Pain is constant and is dull aching. It interferes with sleep
- Grating, popping sensation and crepitus may be felt or heard.

Late

- Decrease in the functional activity like doing simple everyday tasks like using a screw driver, turning a door knob
- Muscle wasting of the forearm.

Investigations

- Plain X-ray
- Laboratory investigations
- MRI.

Procedures

- Position: Supine position with the arm fully adducted by the patient's side and the elbow flexed slightly and the palm resting on a folded towel
- Drugs: 1.5 ml of local anaesthetic and 40 mg of Methylprednisolone
- Syringe: 5 ml/1 inch length/25-gauge.

Techniques

- Paint and drape the area
- Identify the ulnar styloid process
- Identify the inferior radioulnar joint medially at one third distance across the wrist. Mark this point.
- Another easy way to identify the joint is to gently glide distal radius and ulna together
- At the designated point insert the needle and redirect it more medially
- Gently inject the contents into the joint space.

Resistance vs Inference

- More resistance: The needle is within the tendon or ligament. Advance the needle further and inject
- Little resistance: Congratulations you have hit the right spot.

After Care

At the injection site, after the injection

- Apply icepacks
- Apply a firm sterile bandage under pressure.

Complications

- Infection (hence follow strict aseptic measures)
- Transient increase of pain (seen in 25% of the cases)
- Ecchymosis
- Haematoma formation.

Note: The incidence of ecchymosis and haematoma formation can be reduced if immediately after the injection, a firm sterile pressure bandage is applied.

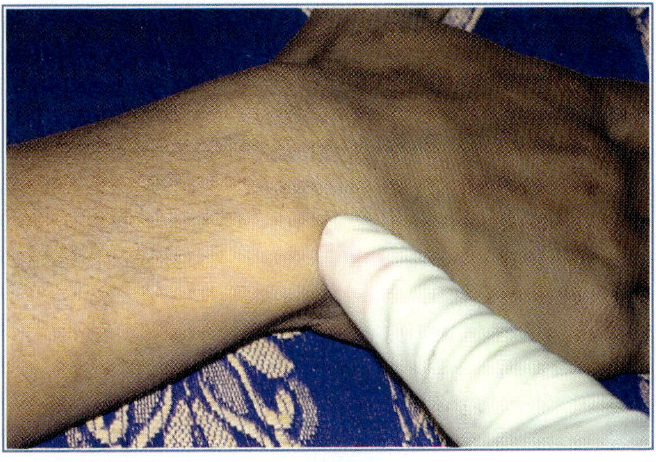

Fig. 2.23A: Identify the ulnar styloid process and mark it

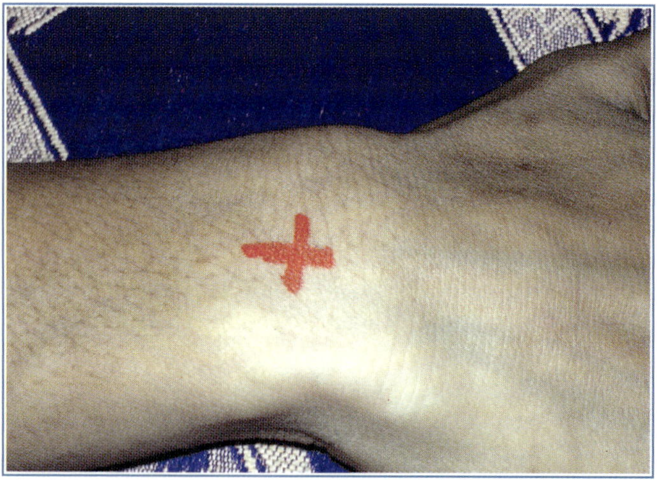

Fig. 2.23B: Identify the inferior ulnar joint medially to this point

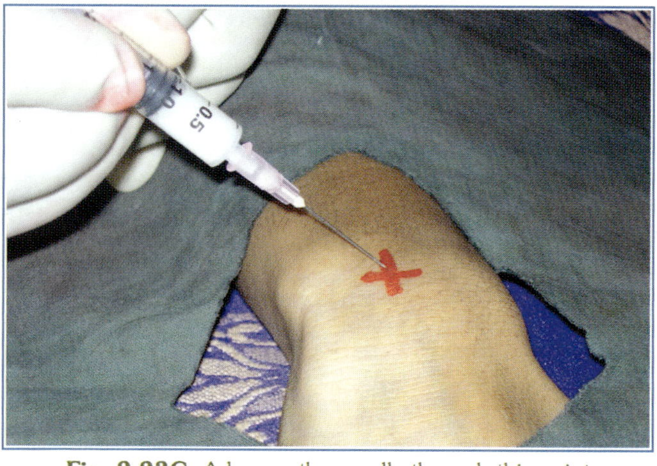

Fig. 2.23C: Advance the needle through this point

Vital facts: Strictly observe the following after the injection:
- Simple analgesics and NSAIDs are advised
- To prevent the exacerbation of pain, avoid heat and gentle range of motion exercises for few days
- Avoid vigorous exercises for few days to prevent increase in pain.

Local Infiltration for the Soft Tissue Lesions around The Wrist

Carpal Tunnel Syndrome

Carpal tunnel syndrome (CTS) is due to compression of the median nerve as it passes through the carpal tunnel at the wrist.

Causes

- Flexor tenosynovitis
- Rheumatoid arthritis
- Pregnancy
- Amyloidosis
- Malunited Colles' fracture
- Other space occupying lesions.

Presentation

- Pain, numbness, paraesthesiae, associated weakness in the hand and wrist that radiate to the thumb, index, middle and radial half of the ring finger
- There could be radiation proximally into the forearm
- Late untreated progressive cases may show motor weakness and may finally lead to flexion contrtacture of the affected fingers.

Onset

- After repeated wrist movements
- Due to repeated pressure on the wrist (e.g. resting of the wrist on the edge of a computer keyboard)
- Direct trauma to the median nerve.

Findings

- Tenderness over the median nerve at the wrist
- Tinel's sign is positive
- Phalen's sign (Wrist is placed in complete unforced flexion for 30 sec). If it produces features of CTS, then the test is positive
- Loss of sensation in the three fingers
- Wasting of the thenar eminence and weakness of the thumb apposition.

Differential Diagnosis

- *Arthritis of the CMC joint of the thumb*: Here Watson's test is positive and radiographic evidence of arthritis is seen.
- *Cervical radiculopathy:* Neck pain and patient may have reflex, motor and sensory changes. In CTS no reflex changes and all neurological changes are restricted to the distribution of the median nerve
- *Diabetic polyneuropathy*: symmetric involvement on both the hands.

Investigations

- Plain X-ray of the wrist
- EMG
- Blood count
- MRI
- Injection technique—both diagnostic and therapeutic.

Procedures

- Position: Supine with the arm fully adducted at the patient's side and the elbow slightly flexed with the dorsum of the hand resting on the folded towel
- Drugs: 3 ml of local anesthetics and 40 mg of methylprednisolone
- Syringe: 5 ml/ 5/8 inches/25-gauge needle.

Techniques

- Instruct the patient to make a fist and flex the wrist so as to identify the palmaris longus tendon
- Now prepare and drape the skin
- Insert the needle at an angle of 30 degrees just medial to the palmaris longus tendon and proximal to the crease of the wrist
- Advance the needle till the tip is just beyond the tendon
- If you have hit the right spot, a paraesthesia should be felt in the distribution of the median nerve
- If paraesthesia is felt, gently aspiration is done to identify the blood

- If aspiration is negative, and if there is no persistent paraesthesiae, 3 ml of drugs is injected
- If you hit the bone or if no paraesthesia is elicited, withdraw and re-inject.

After Care

At the injection site, after the injection

- Apply icepacks
- Apply a firm sterile bandage under pressure.

Complications

- Infection (hence follow strict aseptic measures)
- Transient increase of pain (seen in 25% of the cases)
- Ecchymosis
- Haematoma formation.

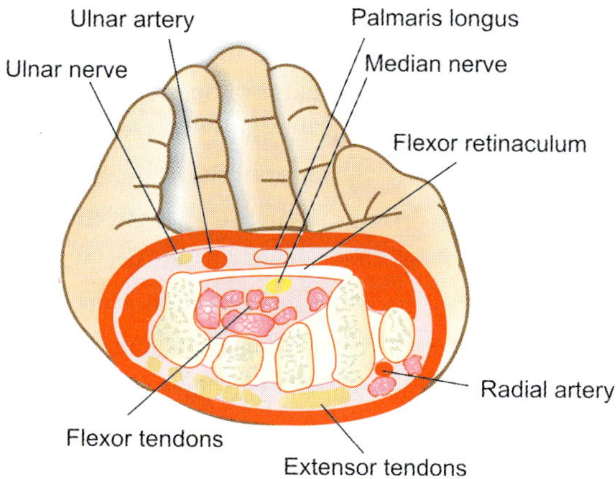

Fig. 2.24A: Anatomy of the carpal tunnel

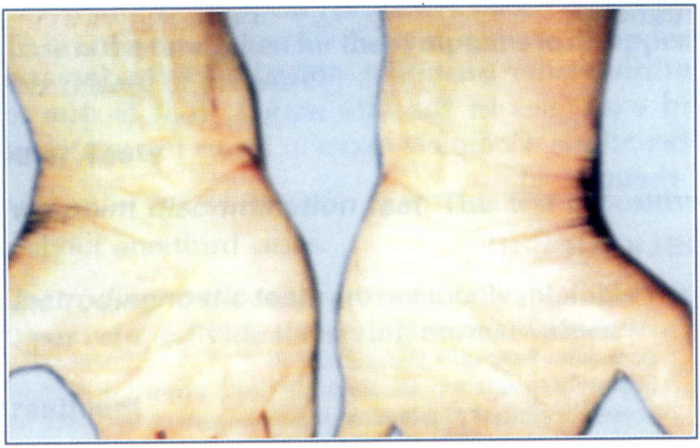

Fig. 2.24B: Clinical photograph of bilateral carpal tunnel syndrome

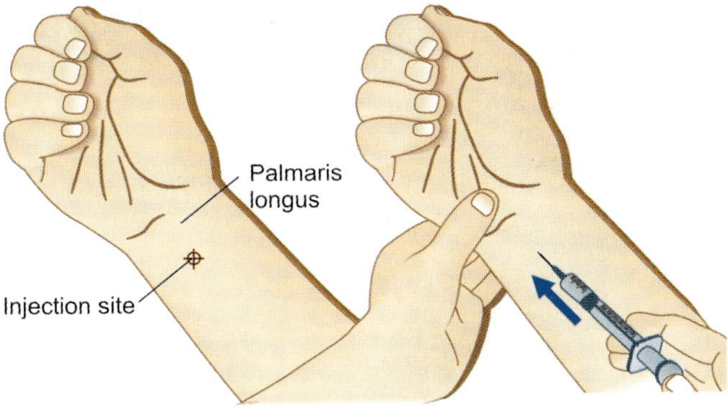

Fig. 2.24C: Pictorial display of injection into the carpal tunnel

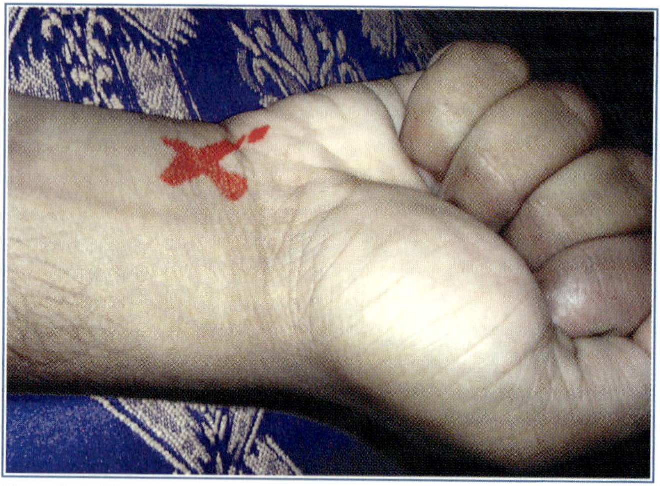

Fig. 2.24D: Instruct the patient to make a fist and flex the wrist so as to identify the palmaris longus tendon

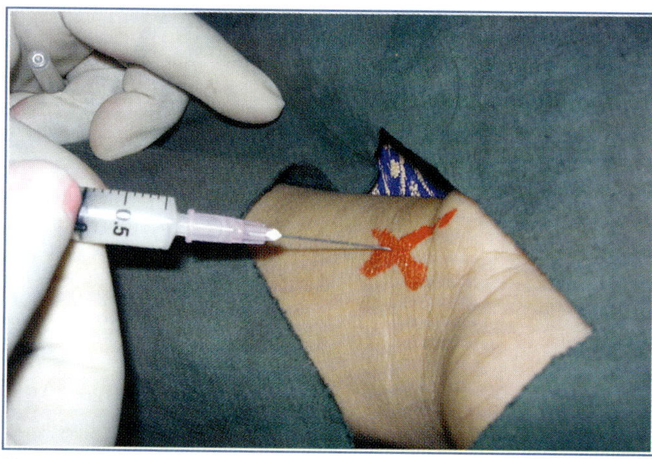

Fig. 2.24E: Insert the needle at an angle of 30 degrees just medial to the palmaris longus tendon and proximal to the crease of the wrist

Note: The incidence of ecchymosis and haematoma formation can be reduced if immediately after the injection, a firm sterile pressure bandage is applied.

Vital facts: Strictly observe the following after the injection:
- Simple analgesics and NSAIDs are advised
- To prevent the exacerbation of pain, avoid heat and gentle range of motion exercises for few days
- Avoid vigorous exercises for few days to prevent increase in pain.

Ulnar Tunnel Syndrome (UTS)

UTS is an entrapment neuropathy of the ulnar nerve as it courses through the Guyon's canal at the wrist.

Causes

- Space occupying lesions
- Ganglion
- Aneurysm of the ulnar artery
- Fractures of the distal ulna and carpals
- Repetitive wrist movements when the hand is used to hammer the hub caps or from handle bar compression during long distance cycling.

Presentation

- The most common presentation is pure motor neuropathy without pain due to compression of the deep palmar branch of the ulnar nerve. There will be painless paralysis of the intrinsic muscles of the hand.

- It could also present mixed sensory and motor neuropathy. It presents as pain, numbness and paraesthesia of the wrist that may radiate to the ulnar aspect of the palm, dorsum of the hand and the little finger and medial half of the ring finger.
- It may also radiate proximally into the forearm.
- The pain worsens in the night and by vigorous movements of the wrist.

Late

- Wasting of the medial half of the hand
- Flexion contracture of the affected fingers.

Findings

- Tenderness over the ulnar nerve at the wrist
- Tinel's sign is positive
- Decreased sensation over the ulnar aspect of the hand, ring finger and entire little finger
- Weakness of the intrinsic muscles of the hand.

Differential Diagnosis

- Arthritis of the CMC joint
- Diabetic polyneuropathy
- Cervical radiculopathy
- Pancoast's tumor compressing the medial cord of the brachial plexus.

Investigations

- Laboratory tests
- Plain X-ray
- MIR
- Injection technique.

Procedures

- Position: Supine with the arm fully adducted at the patient side and the elbow slightly flexed with the dorsum of the hand resting on a folded towel
- Drugs: 3 ml of local anaesthetic and 40 mg of methylprednisolone
- Syringe: 5 ml of 5/8" and 25-gauge needle.

Techniques

- With the patient in the above position, instruct the patient to make a fist and the wrist is simultaneously flexed to identify the flexor carpi ulnaris tendon
- Paint and drape the area
- Now insert the needle just lateral to the tendon at an angle of 30-degree angle just proximal to the crease of the wrist. Advance the needle slowly beyond the tendon
- If paraesthesia is elicited in the distribution of the ulnar nerve, congratulations you are in the right spot. Now slightly withdraw the needle and aspirate for blood
- If aspiration test is negative and if there is no persistent paraesthesiae, inject the contents of the syringe slowly
- If you hit the bone or if no paraesthesia is elicited, withdraw the needle and inject the contents of the syringe.

After Care

At the injection site, after the injection

- Apply icepacks
- Apply a firm sterile bandage under pressure.

Complications

- Infection (hence follow strict aseptic measures)
- Transient increase of pain (seen in 25% of the cases)
- Inadvertent injection into the ulnar nerve
- Persistent paraesthesiae
- Since Guyon's canal is a closed space there contents have to be injected slowly to avoid pressure effects
- Ecchymosis
- Haematoma formation.

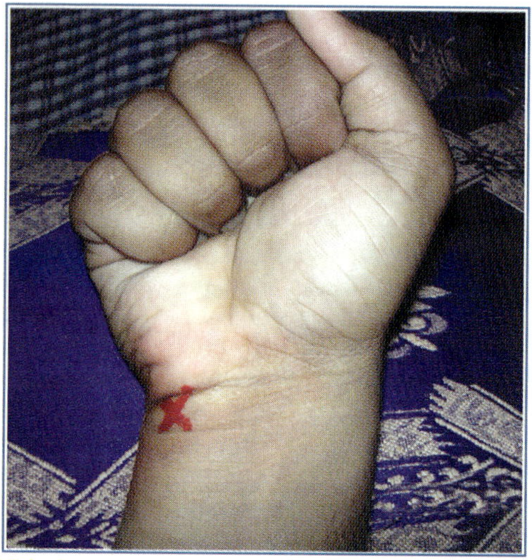

Fig. 2.25A: Instruct the patient to make a fist and flex the wrist ulnarwards so as to identify the flexor carpi ulnaris tendon

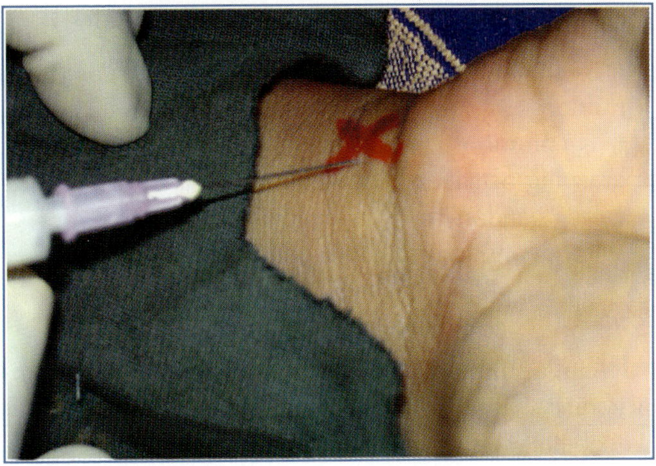

Fig. 2.25B: Insert the needle at an angle of 30 degrees just lateral to the tendon and proximal to the crease of the wrist

Note: The incidence of ecchymosis and haematoma formation can be reduced if immediately after the injection, a firm sterile pressure bandage is applied.

Vital facts: Strictly observe the following after the injection:

- Simple analgesics and NSAIDs are advised
- To prevent the exacerbation of pain, avoid heat and gentle range of motion exercises for few days
- Avoid vigorous exercises for few days to prevent increase in pain.

De Quervain's Tenosynovitis

It is a tenosynovitis of the tendons of the abductor pollicis longus and extensor pollicis brevis at the level of the styloid process.

Causes

- It is mainly due to trauma following repetitive twisting motions
- It is common in people engaged in repetitive hand grasping activities like politicians shaking hands, ice-cream vendors scooping icecreams, etc.
- Without any trauma in pregnant ladies.

Course

If the inflammation becomes chronic there could be thickening of the tendon sheaths leading to constriction this sheath. This could leads to a lock thumb or trigger thumb.

Features

- Pain is localized to the region of the radial styloid process
- It is constant and increases with active pinching activities of the thumb or ulnar deviation of the wrist
- Patient complains of inability to hold a coffee cup or turn a screw driver
- Sleep disturbance is common
- Tenderness along the distal radius and swelling over the tendon sheaths
- There is a point tenderness over the radial styloid
- There could be a creaking sensation due to flexion and extension of the thumb
- Thumb range of movements could be reduced
- Trigger thumb is a possibility
- Finkelstein's test is positive.

Differential Diagnosis

- Entrapment of the lateral ante brachial cutaneous nerve
- Arthritis of the first CMC joints
- Gout
- Cheralgia Paraesthetica
- C 6-7 radiculopathy.

Investigations

- Plain X-ray of the wrist
- MRI
- Laboratory investigations
- EMG studies
- Injection method.

Procedures

- Position: Supine with the arm fully adducted at the patients side and the ulnar surface of the wrist and hand resting on a folded towel to relax the affected tendons
- Drugs: 2 ml of local anaesthetic and 40 mg of methylprednisolone
- Syringe: 5 ml/1 inch/25 or 27-gauge needle.

Techniques

- Put the patient in the above position with the thumb maximally abducted
- Insert the needle at an angle of 45 degrees towards the radial styloid process inbetween the two tendons

- If you hit the bone withdraw the needle. Now inject the contents of the syringe in a proximal direction
- If there is resistance the needle could be in the tendon or ligament. Withdraw and re-inject.
- If you have hit the right spot there will be little resistance to the injection.

After Care

At the injection site, after the injection

- Apply icepacks
- Apply a firm sterile bandage under pressure.

Complications

- Rupture of the tendon if wrongly injected
- Infection (hence follow strict aseptic measures)
- Transient increase of pain (seen in 25% of the cases)
- Ecchymosis
- Haematoma formation
- Injury to sensory branch of the radial nerve.

Note: The incidence of ecchymosis and haematoma formation can be reduced if immediately after the injection, a firm sterile pressure bandage is applied.

Vital facts: Strictly observe the following after the injection:

- Simple analgesics and NSAIDs are advised
- To prevent the exacerbation of pain, avoid heat and gentle range of motion exercises for few days
- Avoid vigorous exercises for few days to prevent increase in pain.

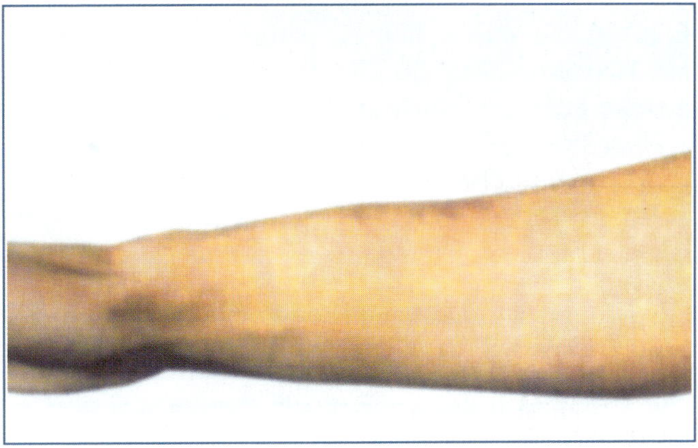

Fig. 2.26A: Clinical photograph of the De Quervain's disease

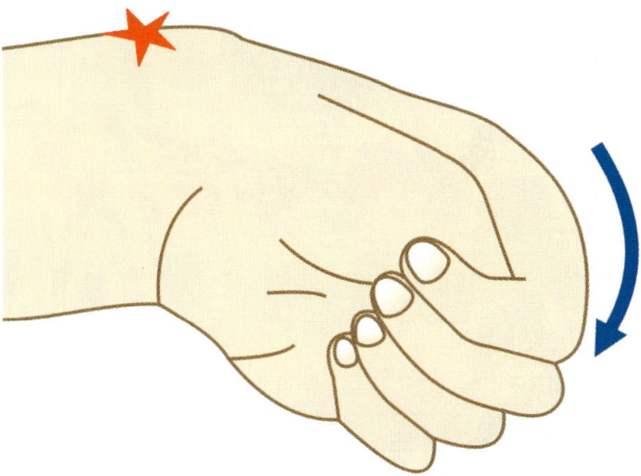

Fig. 2.26B: Method of performing the Finkelstein's test

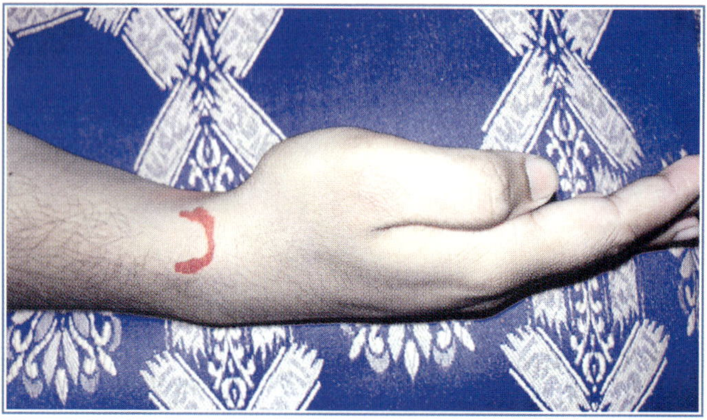

Fig. 2.26C: Identify the radial styloid process and mark it with a sterile marker

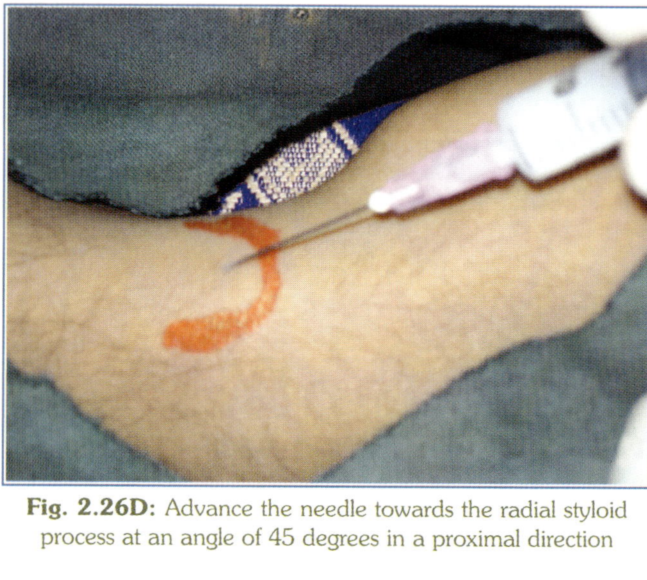

Fig. 2.26D: Advance the needle towards the radial styloid process at an angle of 45 degrees in a proximal direction

GANGLION

Ganglion is herniation of the synovial tissues from joint capsules or tendon sheaths. Due to irritation following friction it produces increased amounts of synovial fluid, which gets collected in cyst like cavities producing prominent, swelling over the dorsum of the wrist.

Due to one way valve phenomenon, the cyst expands in size and the fluid cannot flow freely back into the synovial cavity.

Presentation

- Pain over the wrist. It increases with extreme flexion and extension
- Pain is constant and dull aching
- Swelling which is unsightly often brings the patient to the doctor. It is smooth to palpate and tranilluminates
- Palpation causes pain.

Investigations

- Laboratory tests
- Plain X-ray of the wrist
- MRI
- Ultrasonography.

Note: Ganglion usually arises from the joint space of the lunate or from the tendon of extensor carpi radialis.

Procedures

- Position: Supine with the arm fully adducted at the patients side and the elbow is slightly flexed with the palm of the hand resting on a folded towel.

- Drugs: 1.5 ml local anaesthetics and 40 mg methylprednisolone
- Syringe: 5 ml/1 inch/22-gauge needle.

Techniques

- Patient is in the position mentioned above
- The area is prepared and draped
- The needle is inserted in the center of the ganglion and the contents are aspirated
- After the aspiration, the contents of the syringe is slowly injected
- There should be little resistance to the infection
- The needle is removed and pressure bandage is applied.

Caution

If during the aspiration bone is encountered, the needle is withdrawn back into the cyst and gentle aspiration is carried out.

After Care

At the injection site, after the injection

- Apply icepacks
- Apply a firm sterile bandage under pressure.

Complications

- Infection (hence follow strict aseptic measures)
- Transient increase of pain (seen in 25% of the cases)

- Ecchymosis
- Haematoma formation.

Note: The incidence of ecchymosis and haematoma formation can be reduced if immediately after the injection, a firm sterile pressure bandage is applied.

Vital facts: Strictly observe the following after the injection:
- Simple analgesics and NSAIDs are advised
- To prevent the exacerbation of pain, avoid heat and gentle range of motion exercises for few days
- Avoid vigorous exercises for few days to prevent increase in pain.

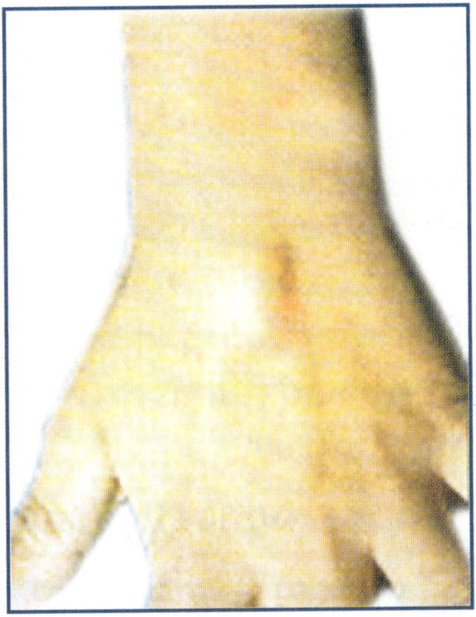

Fig. 2.27A: Clinical photograph of a ganglion on the dorsum of the wrist

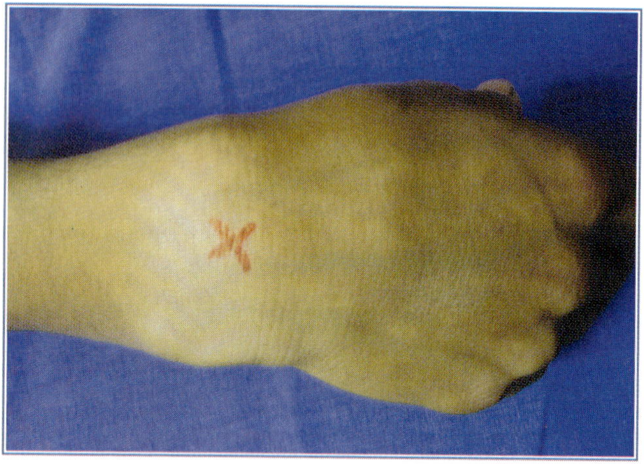

Fig. 2.27B: Mark the center of the ganglion

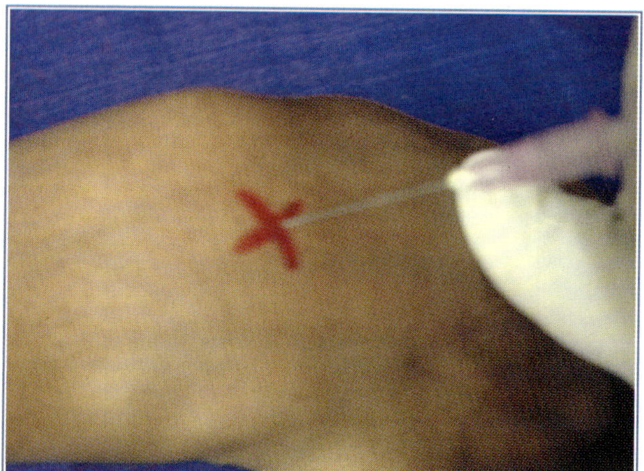

Fig. 2.27C: The needle for the aspiration should be inserted straight into the center of the ganglion

HAND

Dupuytren's Contracture

It is a progressive fibrosis of the palmar fascia. As the disease progresses it involves the flexor tendons of the hand. This results in flexion contractures of the hand. The ring and little fingers are more commonly affected.

Note: As the disease progresses, the pain may burn out but contractures may lead to permanent deformity of the fingers.

Causes

- Genetic basis
- Repetitive trauma to the palm
- Diabetes
- Alcoholism
- Chronic barbiturate use.

Presentation

- Initially hard, fibrotic nodules may be palpated along the flexor tendons
- Pain may be present
- Later taut fibrous bands develop and may cross the metacarpophalangeal and the proximal interphalangeal joints. These are not painful.
- Finger extension is limited though finger flexion remains normal
- Hand functions are severely affected.

Investigations

- Plain X-ray of the hand
- Laboratory investigations
- MRI.

Procedures

- Position: Same as in for the trigger finger
- Drugs: 2 ml of local anesthetics and 40 mg of Methylprednisolone
- Syringes: 5 ml/1 inch/25-gauge needle.

Techniques

- Patient is put in the above position
- Paint and drape the area
- Just lateral to the fibrosis, the needle is inserted at an angle of 45 degree and parallel to the fibrosis
- The contents are slowly injected. Some resistance to the injection is expected due to fibrosis of the surrounding tissues. But if there is significant resistance, the needle could be in the tendon or fibrotic nodule. Withdraw and re-inject
- If you hit the bone, withdraw redirect and inject.

After Care

At the injection site, after the injection

- Apply icepacks
- Apply a firm sterile bandage under pressure.

Complications

- Infection (hence follow strict aseptic measures)
- Transient increase of pain (seen in 25% of the cases)
- Ecchymosis
- Haematoma formation.

Note: The incidence of ecchymosis and haematoma formation can be reduced if immediately after the injection, a firm sterile pressure bandage is applied.

Vital facts: Strictly observe the following after the injection:
- Simple analgesics and NSAIDs are advised
- To prevent the exacerbation of pain, avoid heat and gentle range of motion exercises for few days
- Avoid vigorous exercises for few days to prevent increase in pain.

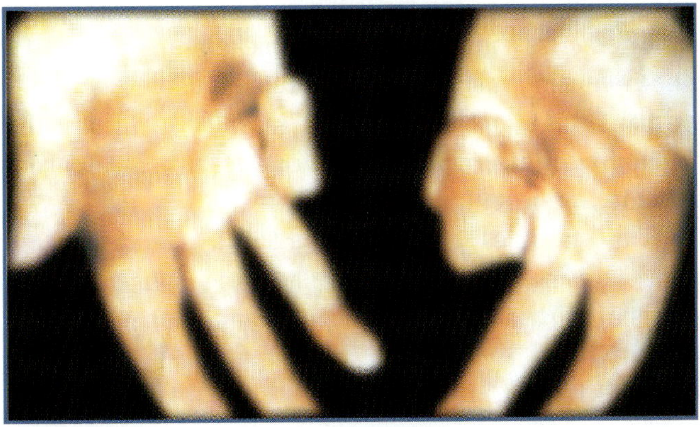

Fig. 2.28A: Clinical photograph of bilateral Dupuytren's contracture

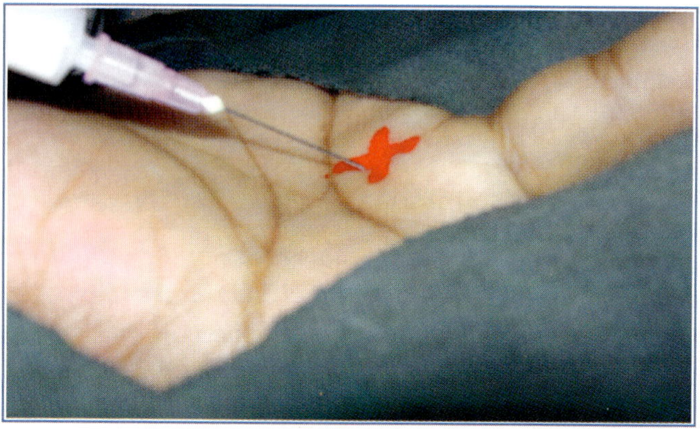

Fig. 2.28B: The needle should be inserted at an angle of 45 degrees just parallel to the fibrosis

Trigger Finger Syndrome

In trigger finger syndrome there is inflammation and swelling of the tendons of the flexor digitorum superficialis. If this becomes chronic it results in thickening of the tendon sheath causing it's constriction. Repetitive gliding of the tendons through the narrow sheath results in the development of nodules over it due to repetitive chronic pressure and irritation.

These nodules may get caught in the tendon sheath under a restraining pulley when it passes over them. This results in triggering or locking phenomena.

Causes

- Due to repetitive trauma to the tendons
- Due to compression by the heads of the metacarpal bones

- Due to compression by sesamoid bones in this region
- Co-existent arthritis and gout involving the hand may cause or exacerbate the problem
- Commonly seen in people engaged in repetitive hand clenching activities, e.g. gripping a steering wheel or holding a horses reins too tightly.

Presentation

- Pain in the distal palm. It is constant and interferes with sleep. It is increased with active hand gripping activities
- Finger stiffness is often a common complaint
- Many a times patient complains of awakening in the morning with the fingers locked in flexed position during sleep
- Tender nodules may be palpated over the tendon with maximum tenderness over the heads of the metacarpal bones. These nodules are usually over the flexor digitorum superficialis
- There is decrease in the finger range of movements
- There are frequent complaints of triggering.

Investigastions

- Laboratory tests:
- Plain X-rays of the hand
- MRI: if joint instability's suspected
- Injection techniques: both diagnostic and therapeutic.

Procedures

- Position: Supine with arm fully adducted at the patient's side and with the distal surface of the hand resting on the folded towel
- Drugs: 2 ml of local anaesthetic and 40 mg of methylprednisolone
- Syringe: 5 ml/1 inch/25-gauge needle.

Techniques

- Identify the affected tendon and the head of the metacarpal beneath
- Prepare and drape the area
- Insert the needle at an angle of 45 degrees to the tendon and proceed parallel to the tendon
- If you hit the bone, withdraw the needle slightly
- Inject the contents of the syringe gently
- If there is little resistance and if the tendon sheath distends after the injection, congratulations, you are bang on target
- If there is significant resistance needle is probably within the tendon. Slightly withdraw and re-inject.

After care

At the injection site, after the injection

- Apply icepacks
- Apply a firm sterile bandage under pressure

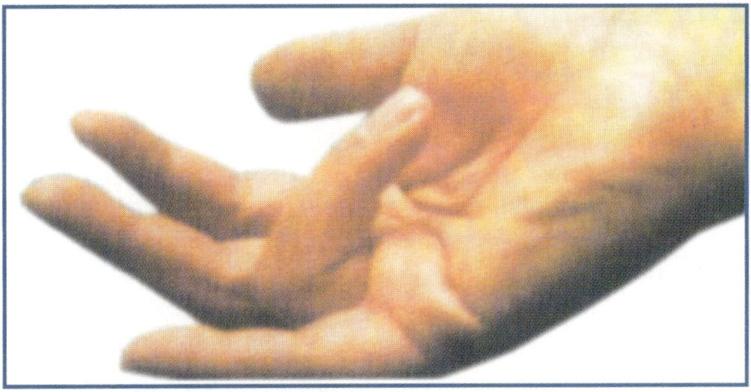

Fig. 2.29A: Clinical photograph of a trigger finger

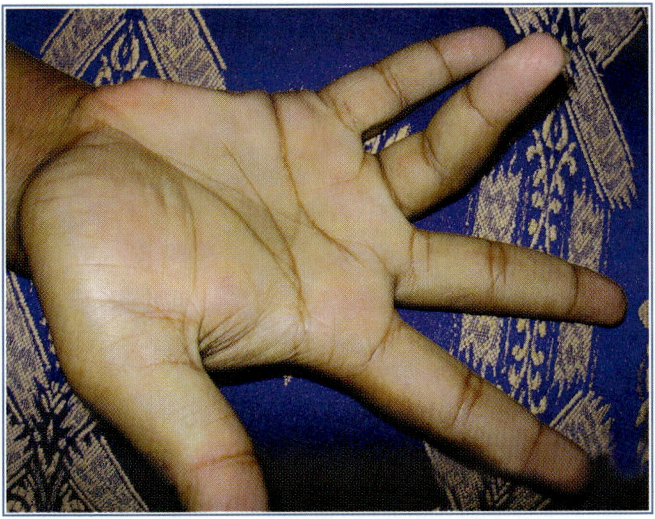

Fig. 2.29B: Identify the affected tendon and the head of the metacarpal bone beneath

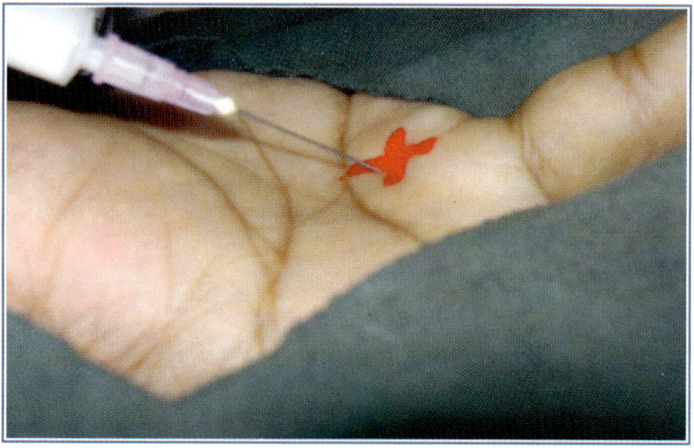

Fig. 2.29C: Insert the needle at an angle of 45 degree to the tendon and proceed parallel to the tendon

Complications

- Infection (hence follow strict aseptic measures)
- Transient increase of pain (seen in 25% of the cases)
- Ecchymosis
- Haematoma formation.

Note: The incidence of ecchymosis and haematoma formation can be reduced if immediately after the injection, a firm sterile pressure bandage is applied.

Vital facts: Strictly observe the following after the injection:
- Simple analgesics and NSAIDs are advised
- To prevent the exacerbation of pain, avoid heat and gentle range of motion exercises for few days
- Avoid vigorous exercises for few days to prevent increase in pain.

Section 3

Injection Techniques in the Trunk and Back

CHEST COMPLEX

SOFT TISSUE LESIONS AROUND THE CHEST

Costosternal Syndrome

Causes

- Osteoarthritis
- Rheumatoid arthritis
- Ankylosing spondylitis
- Reiter's syndrome
- Psoriatic arthritis
- Injuries
- Acceleration and deceleration injuries
- Blunt trauma to the chest
- Subluxation or dislocation
- Overuse or misuse
- Invasion by tumor—primary or secondary malignancies.

Presentation

- Pain in the costosternal area
- Pain increases by active protraction or retraction of the shoulder
- Pain increases by deep inspiration
- Pain increases by full elevation of the arm
- Shrugging of the shoulder increases pain
- Patient keeps the shoulder stiff in neutral position
- Coughing may be difficult

- Costosternal joints and adjacent intercostal muscle are tender to palpation
- There could be a feeling of clicking sensation with movements of the joint.

Investigations

- Laboratory tests
- Plain X-ray of the chest
- MRI
- Injection technique.

Procedures

- Position: Supine
- Drugs: 1 ml of 0.25 per cent preservative free bupivacaine and 40 mg of methylprednisolone
- Syringe: 2 ml/1 ½ inches/ 25-gauge needle.

Techniques

- In the position mentioned above, the point is painted and draped
- Identify the costovertebral joints by careful palpation. Costosternal area is seen easily as a slight bulge at the point where the rib attaches to the sternum
- Insert the needle close to the joint in a slightly medial and a cephalad direction
- If you hit the bone, withdraw the needle and redirect it more medially
- Inject the contents of the syringe gently
- Repeat the procedure for each affected joint.

Resistance vs Inference

- If there is limited resistance, congratulations, you have hit the right spot
- If there is significant resistance, sorry, you are in the wrong space. Withdraw the needle, redirect and inject.

After Care

At the injection site, after the injection

- Apply icepacks
- Apply a firm sterile bandage under pressure.

Complications

- Infection (hence follow strict aseptic measures)
- Transient increase of pain (seen in 25% of the cases)

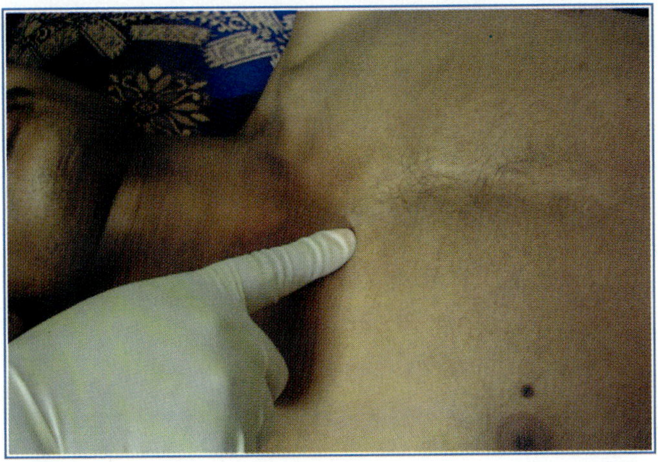

Fig. 3.1A: Identify the costo-vertebral joint by careful palpation

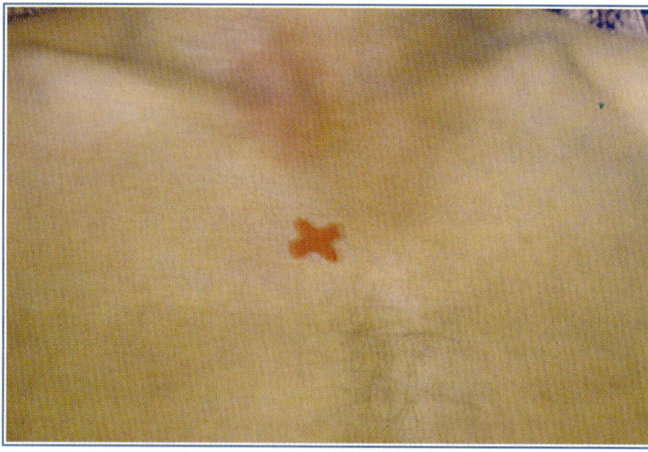

Fig. 3.1B: Mark that point with a sterile marker

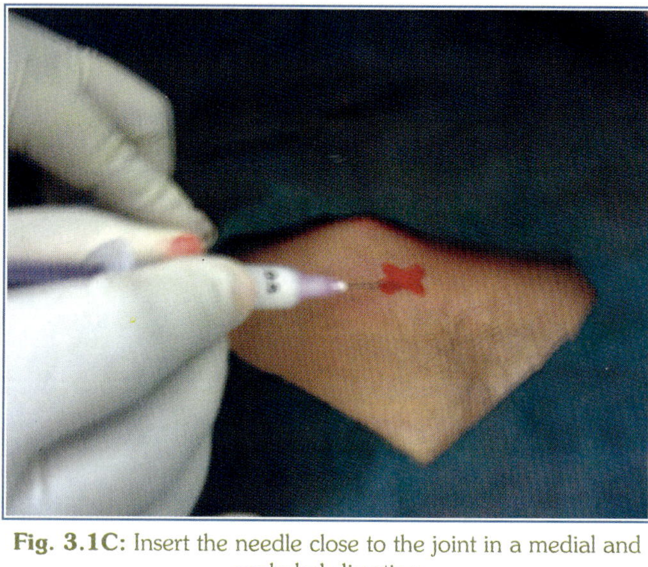

Fig. 3.1C: Insert the needle close to the joint in a medial and cephalad direction

- Ecchymosis
- Haematoma formation

Note: The incidence of ecchymosis and haematoma formation can be reduced if immediately after the injection, a firm sterile pressure bandage is applied

Vital facts: Strictly observe the following after the injection:
- Simple analgesics and NSAIDs are advised
- To prevent the exacerbation of pain, avoid heat and gentle range of motion exercises for few days
- Avoid vigorous exercises for few days to prevent increase in pain.

Tietze's Syndrome

This is characterized by the following:
- It was first described in 1921
- Acute painful swelling of the costal cartilages
- 2nd and 3rd costal cartilages are more commonly involved
- It occurs in the second and third decades (costosternal syndrome occurs only in the 4th decade)
- The onset is usually acute
- It may be associated with concurrent viral upper respiratory tract infections.

Causes

- Microtrauma due to severe coughing or from heavy labor
- Osteoarthritis

- Rheumatoid arthritis
- Ankylosing spondylitis
- Reiter's syndrome
- Psoriatic arthritis
- Accelerretation and deceleration injuries
- Blunt trauma to the chest
- Tumor invasion—primary or secondary.

Presentation

- Pain increases on protraction and retraction of the shoulder, elevation of the shoulder, shrugging, deep inspiration, etc. Cough also increases the pain
- 2nd and 3rd costosternal joints are tender to palpate
- Clicking sensation with movement of the joint.

Investigations

- Laboratory tests
- Plain X-ray of the chest
- MRI
- Injection techniques.

Procedures

- Position: Supine
- Drugs: 1 ml of 0.25 per cent preservative free bupivacaine and 40 mg of methylprednisolone
- Syringe: 2 ml/1 ½ inches/ 25-gauge needle.

Techniques

- In the position mentioned above, the part is painted and draped
- Identify the 2nd and 3rd costosternal joints by careful palpation. Costosternal area is seen easily as a slight bulge at the point where the rib attaches to the sternum
- Insert the needle close to the joint in a slightly medial and a cephalad direction
- If you hit the bone, withdraw the needle and redirect it more medially
- Inject the contents of the syringe gently
- Repeat the procedure for the other affected joint, if any.

Resistance vs Inference

- *If there is limited resistance,* congratulations, you have hit the right spot
- *If there is significant resistance,* sorry, you are in the wrong space. Withdraw the needle, redirect and inject.

After Care

At the injection site, after the injection

- Apply icepacks
- Apply a firm sterile bandage under pressure.

Complications

- Infection (hence follow strict aseptic measures)
- Transient increase of pain (seen in 25% of the cases)

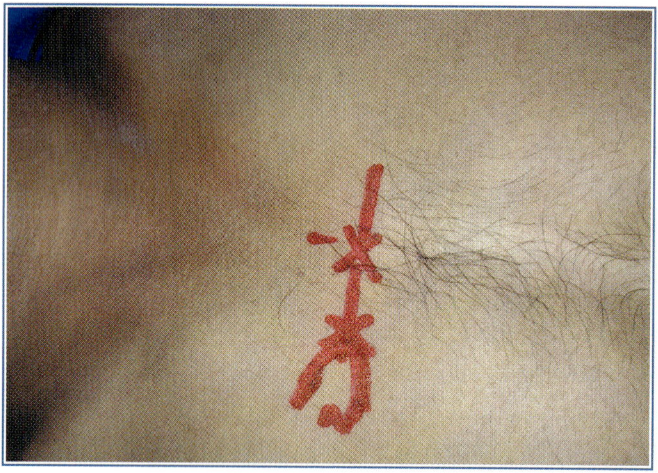

Fig. 3.2A: Mark the sternal angle and label it as 1. Mark the second costochondral junction which is the site of pain in Tietze's syndrome and label it as 2

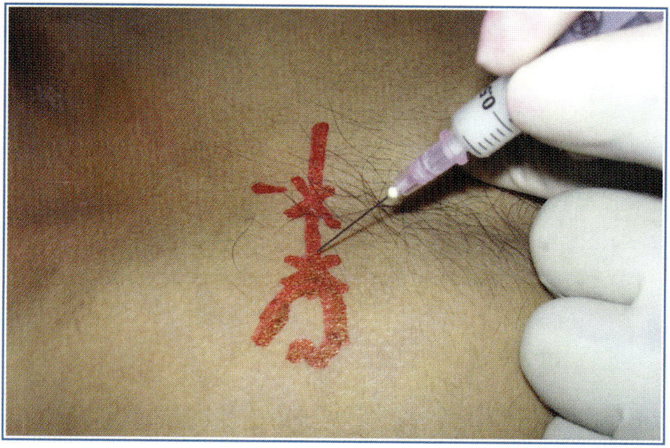

Fig. 3.2B: Inject into the second costochondral junction

- Ecchymosis
- Haematoma formation

Note: The incidence of ecchymosis and haematoma formation can be reduced if immediately after the injection, a firm sterile pressure bandage is applied.

Vital facts: Strictly observe the following after the injection:
- Simple analgesics and NSAIDs are advised
- To prevent the exacerbation of pain, avoid heat and gentle range of motion exercises for few days
- Avoid vigorous exercises for few days to prevent increase in pain.

Manubriosternal Joint Pain Syndrome

Manubriosternal joint pain syndrome mimics the pain of a cardiac origin and may send the alarm bells ringing.

Causes

- Osteoarthritis
- Rheumatoid arthritis
- Ankylosing spondylitis
- Reiter's syndrome
- Psoriatic arthritis
- Acceleration and deceleration injuries
- Blunt trauma to the chest
- Overuse and misuse injuries
- Tumor invasion—primary or secondary.

Presentation

- Pain increases on protraction and retraction of the shoulder, elevation of the shoulder, shrugging, deep inspiration, etc. Cough also increases the pain
- The patient holds the shoulder stiff in neutral position
- Manubriosternal joint is tender to palpate
- If the joint is acutely inflamed, there may be swelling and warmth
- Clicking sensation with movement of the joint.

Investigations

- Laboratory tests—include CBC, ESR, ANA, and PSA tests
- Plain X-ray of the Chest—to rule out any occult bony pathologies
- MRI—is indicated if there is joint instability
- Injection technique is both diagnostic and therapeutic.

Procedures

- Position: Supine
- Drugs: 1 ml of 0,25 per cent preservative free bupivacaine and 40 mg of methylprednisolone
- Syringe: 2 ml/1 ½ inches/ 25-gauge needle.

Techniques

- In the position mentioned above, the part is painted and draped
- Identify the angle of the sternum

- The manubriosternal joint should be easily palpable at this point as a slight indentation
- Insert the needle close to the joint in a slightly medial and a cephalad direction
- If you hit the bone, withdraw the needle and redirect it more medially
- Inject the contents of the syringe gently
- Repeat the procedure for the other affected joint, if any.

Resistance vs Inference

- If there is limited resistance, congratulations, you have hit the right spot
- If there is significant resistance, sorry, you are in the wrong space. Withdraw the needle, redirect and inject.

After Care

At the injection site, after the injection

- Apply icepacks
- Apply a firm sterile bandage under pressure.

Complications

- Infection (hence follow strict aseptic measures)
- Transient increase of pain (seen in 25% of the cases)
- Pneumothorax if the needle is placed too deep and lateral
- Injury to the structures behind the manubria
- Ecchymosis
- Haematoma formation.

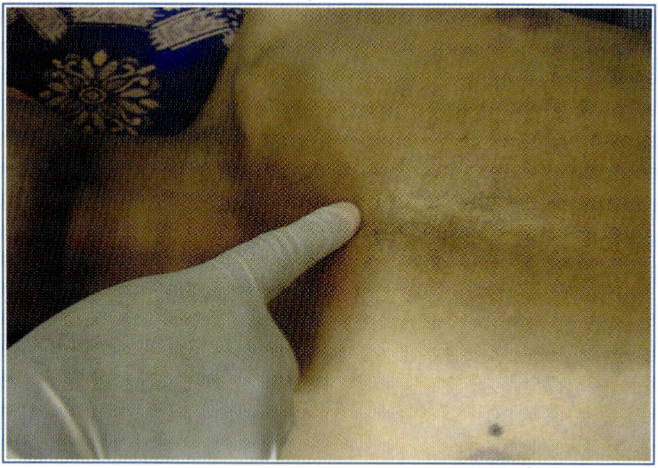

Fig. 3.3A: Identify the angle of the sternum

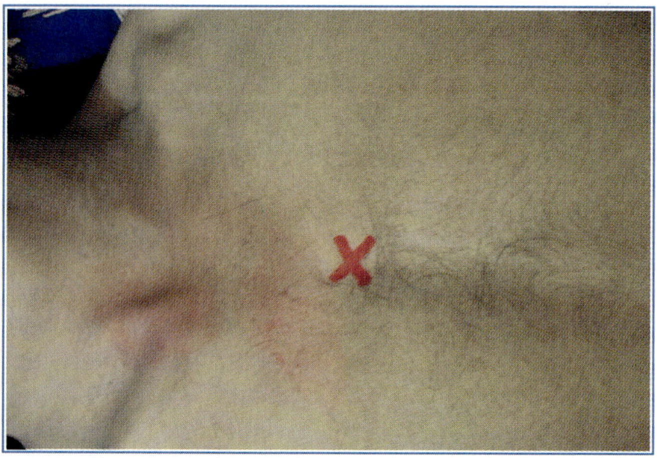

Fig. 3.3B: Now mark the manbriosternal joint

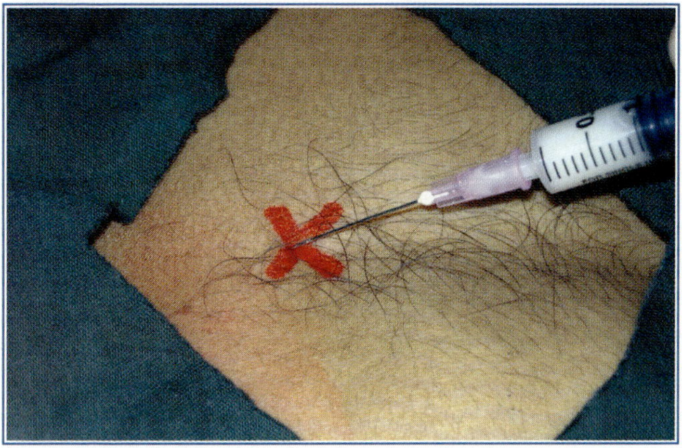

Fig. 3.3C: Insert the needle into the joint in a slightly cephalad direction

Note: The incidence of ecchymosis and haematoma formation can be reduced if immediately after the injection, a firm sterile pressure bandage is applied.

Vital facts: Strictly observe the following after the injection:
- Simple analgesics and NSAIDs are advised
- To prevent the exacerbation of pain, avoid heat and gentle range of motion exercises for few days
- Avoid vigorous exercises for few days to prevent increase in pain.

Sternalis Syndrome

Sternalis muscle lies anterior to the sternal end of the pectoralis major muscle and runs parallel to the sternum. It is however not present in all persons. The pain of sternalis syndrome mimics the pain of a cardiac origin and may send the alarm bells ringing as it may create a fear and panic among the patients as it seems like an heart attack.

It is a myofascial pain syndrome and the trigger points could be found in the midsternal area.

Presentation

- Pain is characteristically located on the midline of the anterior chest wall
- It could radiate to the retrosternal area and also the medial aspect of the arm
- Unlike the pain in costosternal syndrome, here the pain is not increased by movement of the shoulder and the chest wall
- Myofascial trigger points could be felt at the midline over the sternum
- Rarely there could be co-existent trigger points in the pectoralis major muscle and the sternal head of the sternocleidomastoid muscles
- There could trigger points at the lateral border of the scapula too
- Pain is reproduced on palpation of these trigger points and not on the movements of the shoulder or the chest wall
- On stimulation of the trigger point, a positive jump sign is present.

Investigations

- Laboratory tests—this includes CBC,ESR,ANA, and PSA tests

- Plain X-ray of the Chest—to rule out any occult bony pathologies
- MRI—is indicated, if retrosternal mass is suspected
- EMG helps rule out cervical radiculopathy
- Injection technique is both diagnostic and therapeutic.

Procedures

- Position: Supine
- Drugs: 1 ml of 0.25 per cent preservative free bupivacaine and 40 mg of methylprednisolone
- Syringe: 2 ml/1 ½ inches/ 25-gauge needle.

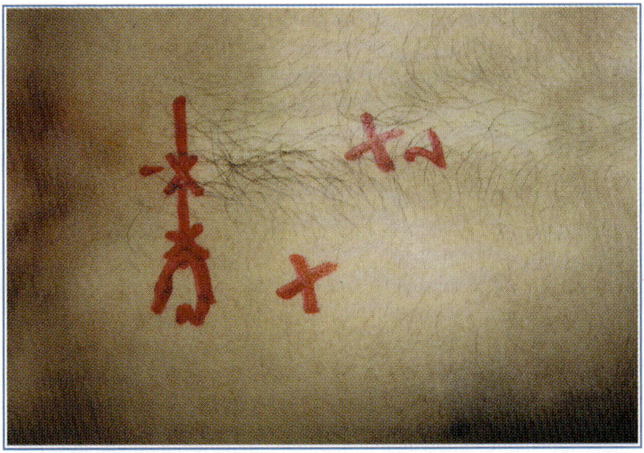

Fig. 3.4A: Identify the sternal angle (Mark 1) and the midline of the sternum (Mark 2)

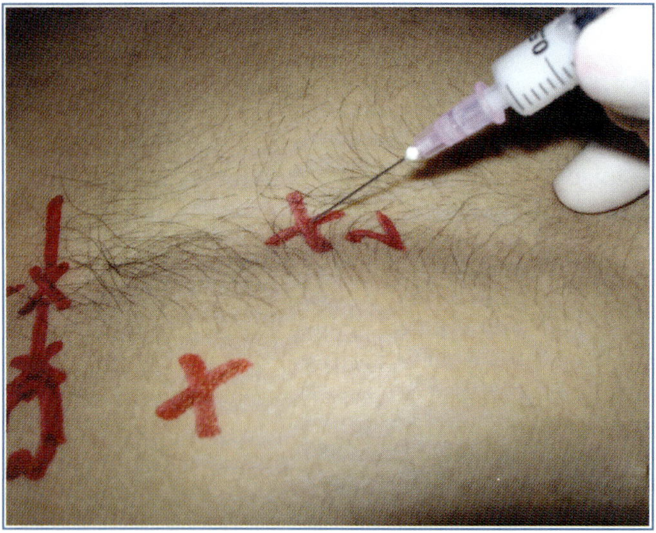

Fig. 3.4B: Inject into the site marked 2

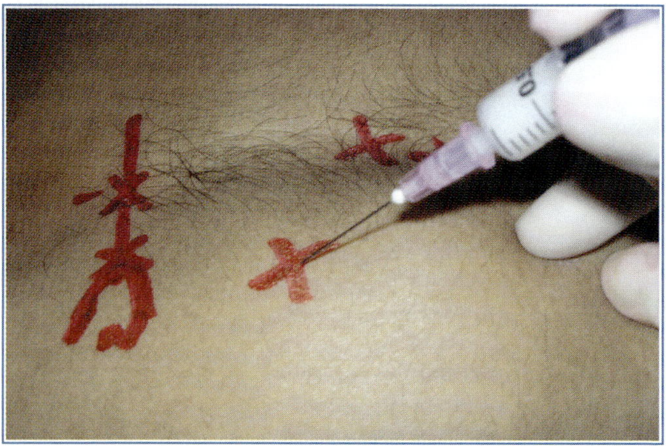

Fig. 3.4C: Inject into the trigger point in the pectoralis major, if present

Techniques

- In the position mentioned above, the part is painted and draped
- Identify the midline of the sternum
- Palpate the sternalis muscle for the trigger points
- On pressing the trigger point a positive jump sign could be elicited
- Mark each trigger point with a sterile marker
- Insert the needle at the center of the trigger point
- Inject the contents of the syringe gently after firmly fixing the needle
- Repeat the procedure for the other trigger points.

Resistance vs Inference

- If there is limited resistance; congratulations, you have hit the right spot
- If there is significant resistance; sorry, you are in the wrong space. Withdraw the needle, redirect and inject.

After Care

At the injection site, after the injection

- Apply icepacks
- Apply a firm sterile bandage under pressure.

Complications

- Infection (hence follow strict aseptic measures)
- Transient increase of pain (seen in 25% of the cases)

- Pneumothorax if the needle is placed too deep and lateral
- Ecchymosis
- Haematoma formation.

Note: The incidence of ecchymosis and haematoma formation can be reduced if immediately after the injection, a firm sterile pressure bandage is applied.

Vital facts: Strictly observe the following after the injection:
- Simple analgesics and NSAIDs are advised
- To prevent the exacerbation of pain, avoid heat and gentle range of motion exercises for few days
- Avoid vigorous exercises for few days to prevent increase in pain.

Xiphodynia Syndrome

Xiphosternal joint pain syndrome mimics the pain of a cardiac and upper abdominal origin and may send the alarm bells ringing.

Causes

- Osteoarthritis
- Rheumatoid arthritis
- Ankylosing spondylitis
- Reiter's syndrome
- Psoriatic arthritis
- Acceleration and deceleration injuries
- Blunt trauma to the chest
- Overuse and misuse injuries
- Tumor invasion—Primary or secondary.

Presentation

- Patient complains of severe intermittent anterior chest wall pain in the region of the xiphoid process
- Pain increases on overeating, bending and stooping
- Coughing may be difficult
- There could be a feeling of nausea
- There may be swelling of the xiphisternal joint
- Xiphosternal joint is tender to palpate
- Clicking sensation with movement of the joint.

Investigations

- Laboratory tests—this includes CBC,ESR,ANA, and PSA tests
- Plain X-ray of the Chest—to rule out any occult bony pathologies
- MRI—is indicated if there is suspicion of any bony occult mass
- Injection technique is both diagnostic and therapeutic.

Procedures

- Position: Supine
- Drugs: 1 ml of 0.25 per cent preservative free bupivacaine and 40 mg of methylprednisolone
- Syringe: 2 ml/1 ½ inches/ 25-gauge needle.

Techniques

- In the position mentioned above, the part is painted and draped

- The xiphosternal joint should be easily palpable as a slight indentation at the point where the xiphoid process attaches to the body of the sternum
- Insert the needle close to the center of the joint in a slight cephalad direction
- If you hit the bone, withdraw the needle and redirect it more medially
- Inject the contents of the syringe gently
- Repeat the procedure for the other affected joint, if any.

Resistance vs Inference

- If there is limited resistance; congratulations, you have hit the right spot
- If there is significant resistance; sorry, you are in the wrong space. Withdraw the needle; redirect and inject.

After Care

At the injection site, after the injection

- Apply icepacks
- Apply a firm sterile bandage under pressure.

Complications

- Infection (hence follow strict aseptic measures)
- Transient increase of pain (seen in 25% of the cases)
- Pneumothorax if the needle is placed too deep and lateral
- Injury to the structures of the mediastinum
- Ecchymosis
- Haematoma formation.

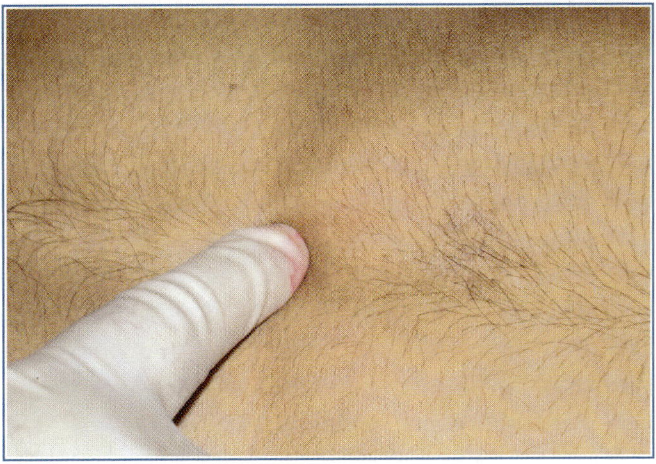

Fig. 3.5A: Identify the xiphisternal joint

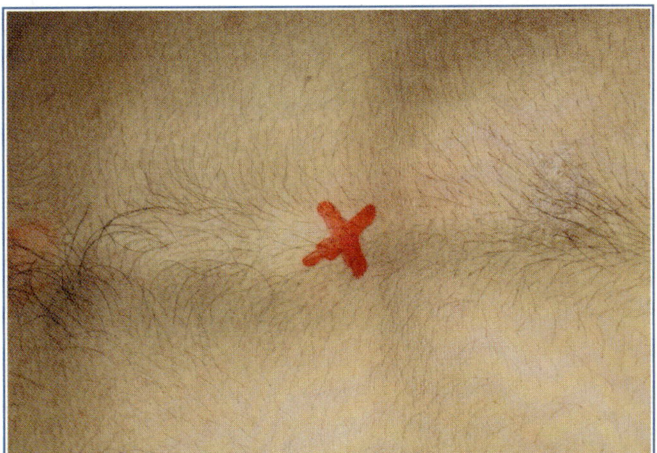

Fig. 3.5B: Mark it with a sterile marker

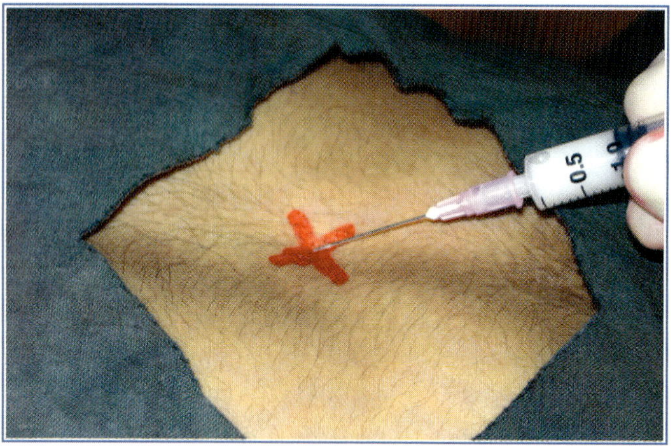

Fig. 3.5C: Insert the needle in the center of the joint in a cephalad direction

Note: The incidence of ecchymosis and haematoma formation can be reduced if immediately after the injection, a firm sterile pressure bandage is applied.

Vital facts: Strictly observe the following after the injection:
- Simple analgesics and NSAIDs are advised
- To prevent the exacerbation of pain, avoid heat and gentle range of motion exercises for few days
- Avoid vigorous exercises for few days to prevent increase in pain.

NECK AND BACK COMPLEX

SOFT TISSUE LESIONS OF THE NECK AND THE BACK

Lumbar Myofascial Pain Syndrome

It is a chronic pain syndrome that affects a focal or regional portion of the body. It is more common in the muscles of the back. The characteristic feature of this condition is the presence of the trigger points in the affected muscles and is the pathognomonic feature.

Causes

- Flexion and extension injuries of the back
- Repeated micro-trauma secondary to improper lifting and bending activities.

Predisposing Factors

- Unaccustomed physical activity
- Poor posture
- Old injuries
- Poor nutritional status
- Psychological or behavioural abnormalities.

Presentation

- Pain in the affected muscles. It is usually referred to other parts of the body
- Pain on the trigger point increases on pressing the point firmly
- Pain increases on stretching.

Signs

- On palpation, taut muscle fibers are identified
- Jump sign: On pressing and releasing the trigger point, patient involuntarily withdraws the affected muscles. This is called the Jump sign.

Note: The trigger point and jump sign are pathgnomonic signs

- Muscle stiffness and fatigue
- Depression and other psychological problems are usually affected.

Procedures

Principles

- Trigger points injections are directed at the primary trigger point and not in the area of the referred pain
- The goal is to block the trigger of the persistent pain
- Prone or lateral position helps prevent vasovagal attack
- Strong asepsis is a must to prevent infection.

Position: Supine

- Drugs: 10 ml of 0.25 per cent preservative free bupivacaine and 40 mg of methylprednisolone
- Syringe: 10 ml/1 ½ inches/ 25-gauge needle.

Techniques

- In the position mentioned above, the point is painted and draped
- Identify the trigger point by careful palpation

- Paint and drape the area
- With a gloved finger reidentify the trigger point
- Insert the needle through the center of the trigger point and inject about 0.5 ml to 1 ml of the solution into each trigger point
- Inject the contents of the syringe gently
- Repeat the procedure for each trigger point
- 2 to 5 injections may be required to abolish the trigger pain.

Resistance vs Inference

- If there is limited resistance: Congratulations, you have hit the right spot
- If there is significant resistance: Sorry, you are in the wrong space. Withdraw the needle, redirect and inject

After Care

At the injection site, after the injection

- Apply icepacks
- Apply a firm sterile bandage under pressure

Complications

- Infection (hence follow strict aseptic measures)
- Transient increase of pain (seen in 25% of the cases)
- Ecchymosis
- Haematoma formation.

Note: The incidence of ecchymosis and haematoma formation can be reduced if immediately after the injection, a firm sterile pressure bandage is applied.

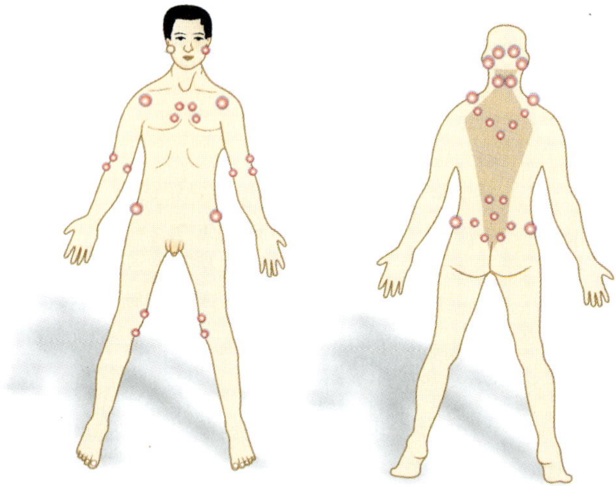

Fig. 3.6A: Site of pain and tenderness in fibromyalgia and lumbar myofascial syndromes

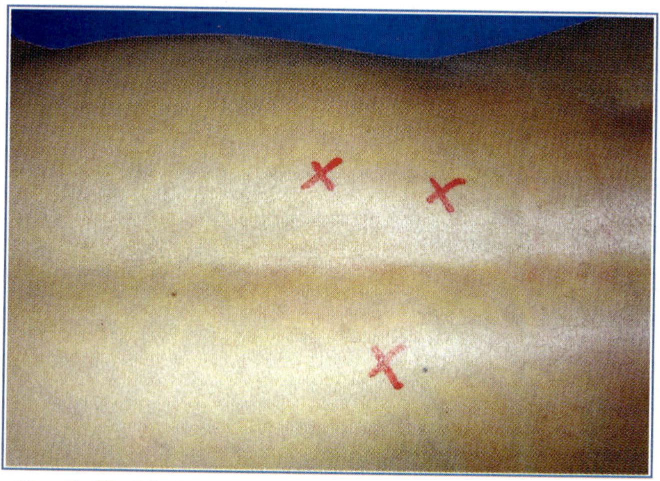

Fig. 3.6B: Mark the points of tenderness in the back muscles

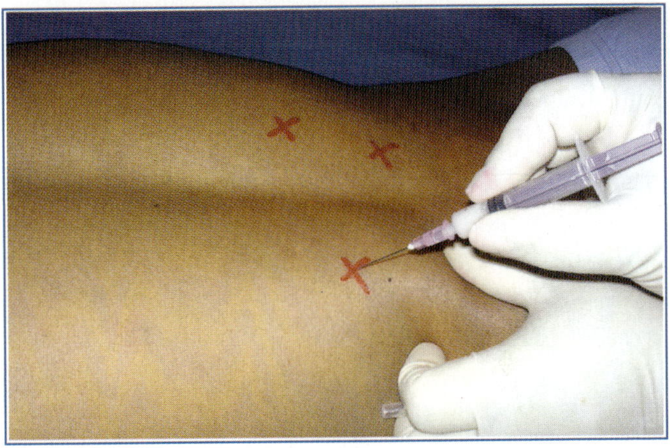

Fig. 3.6C

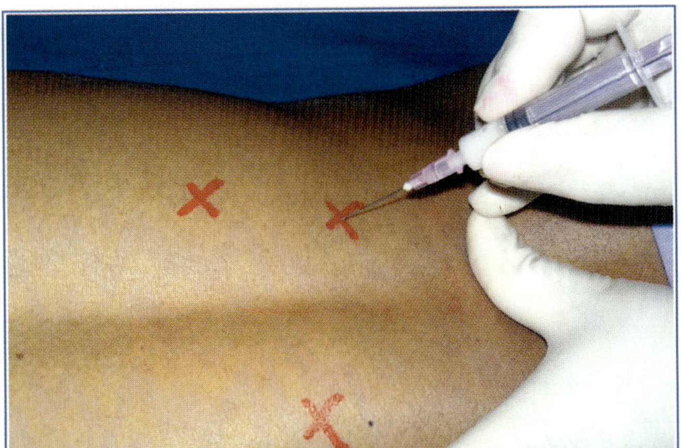

Fig. 3.6D

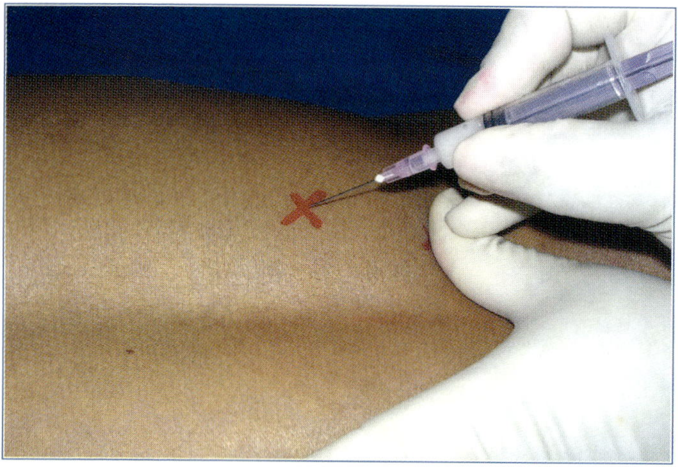

Fig. 3.6E

Figs 3.6C to E: Inject the contents of the syringe into the tender point one by one

Vital facts: Strictly observe the following after the injection:

- Simple analgesics and NSAIDs are advised
- To prevent the exacerbation of pain, avoid heat and gentle range of motion exercises for few days
- Avoid vigorous exercises for few days to prevent increase in pain.

Complications

- Infection
- Ecchymosis
- Haematoma
- Pneumothorax.

Adjunctive treatment: To treat the underlying depression, amitriptyline and nortriptyline single bed time dose of 10 to 25 mg/day is given.

Trapezius Myofascial Pain Syndrome

It is a chronic pain syndrome that affects a focal or regional portion of the body. It is more common in the posterior neck muscles. The characteristic feature of this condition is the presence of the trigger points in the affected muscles and is the pathognomonic features.

Causes

- Flexion and extension injuries of the neck
- Repeated micro-trauma secondary to pressure from the straps of the purse, backpacks, laptops, etc. This leads to the development of trigger points.
- The trapezius muscle is particularly susceptible to the stress induced myofascial pain syndrome.

Predisposing Factors

- Unaccustomed physical activity
- Poor posture
- Old injuries
- Poor nutritional status
- Psychological or behavioral abnormalities
- Chronic stress and depression.

Presentation

- Pain in the affected posterior neck muscles
- It is usually referred to the neck, mastoid region, angle of the jaw and upper extremity
- The patient may believe to have an heart attack
- Pain on the trigger point increases on pressing the point firmly
- Pain increases on stretching
- There could be stiffness and fatigue.

Signs

- On palpation, taut muscle fibers are identified
- On firm pressure over the trigger point there is increase in the local and the referred pain
- Jump sign: On pressing and releasing the trigger point, patient involuntarily withdraws the affected muscles. This is called the Jump sign.

Note: The trigger point and jump sign are pathgnomonic signs.

- Muscle stiffness and fatigue
- Depression and other psychological problems are usually affected.

Procedures

Principles

- Trigger points injections are directed at the primary trigger point and not in the area of the referred pain

- The goal is to block the trigger of the persistent pain
- Prone or lateral position helps prevent vasovagal attack
- Strong asepsis is a must to prevent infection.

Position

- Supine
- Drugs: 10 ml of 0.25 per cent preservative free bupivacaine and 40 mg of methylprednisolone
- Syringe: 10 ml/1 ½ inches/ 25-gauge needle.

Techniques

- In the position mentioned above, the point is painted and draped
- Identify the trigger point by careful palpation
- Paint and drape the area
- With a gloved finger re-identify the trigger point
- Insert the needle through the center of the trigger point and inject about 0.5 ml to 1 ml of the solution into each trigger point
- Inject the contents of the syringe gently
- Repeat the procedure for each trigger point
- 2 to 5 injections maybe required to abolish the trigger pain.

After care: At the injection site, after the injection

- Apply icepacks
- Apply a firm sterile bandage under pressure.

Complications

- Infection (hence follow strict aseptic measures)
- Transient increase of pain (seen in 25% of the cases)

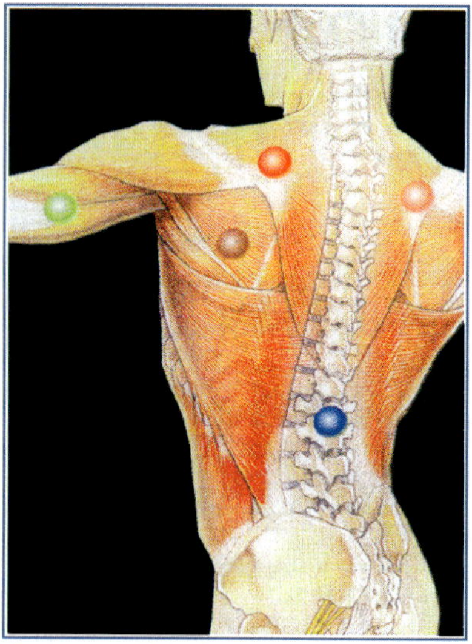

Fig. 3.7A: The point of tendernss in trapezius myofascial pain syndrome

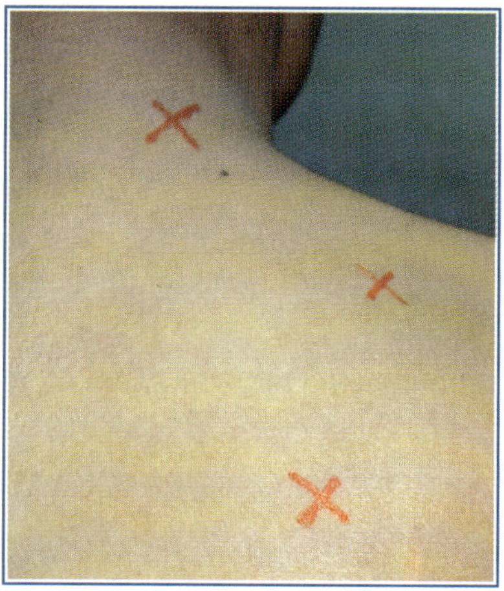

Fig. 3.7B: Mark all the trigger points of pain with a sterile marker

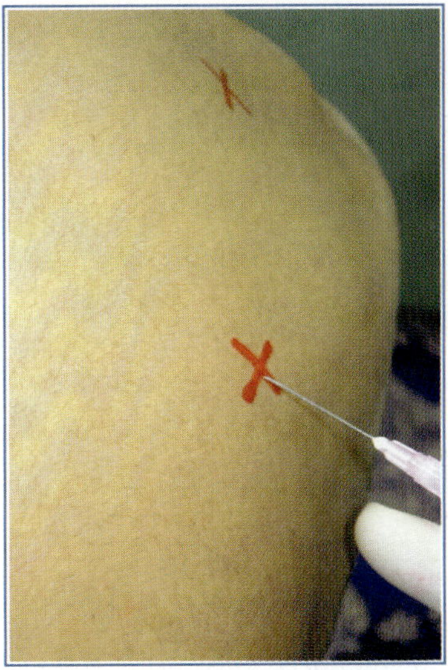

Fig. 3.7C: Injection of the pain point

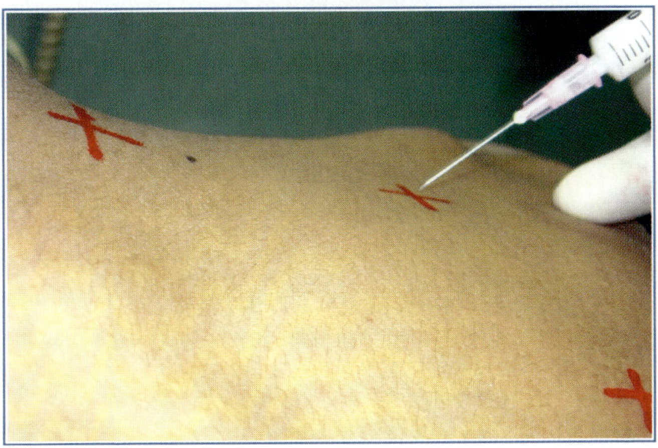

Fig. 3.7D: Injection of the second pain point

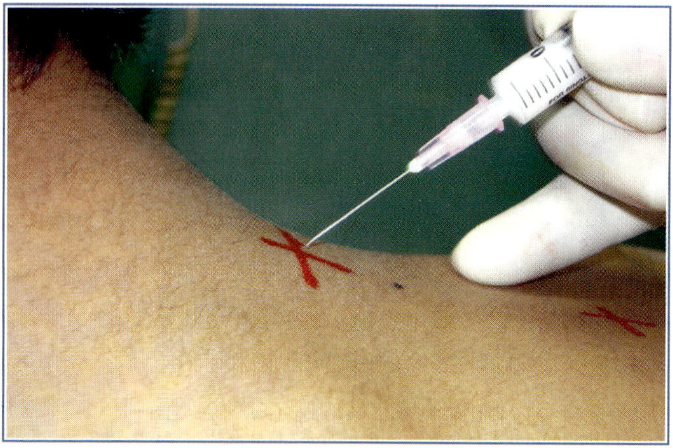

Fig. 3.7E: Injection of the third pain point

- Intravascular injection into the vertebral artery
- This could lead to seizures and ataxia
- Pneumothorax could result due to use of long needles
- Ecchymosis
- Haematoma formation.

Note: The incidence of ecchymosis and haematoma formation can be reduced if immediately after the injection, a firm sterile pressure bandage is applied.

Vital facts: Strictly observe the following after the injection:
- Simple analgesics and NSAIDs are advised
- To prevent the exacerbation of pain, avoid heat and gentle range of motion exercises for few days
- Avoid vigorous exercises for few days to prevent increase in pain.

Adjunctive treatment: To treat the underlying depression, amitriptyline and nortriptyline single bed time dose of 10 to 25 mg/day is given.

INJECTIONS INTO THE SPINE

Injections into the spine are performed for two reasons one is for diagnosis and another is for treatment.

Diagnostic Injections

Injections are called diagnostic when they help locate the source of pain. These are usually referred to as blocks. After anaesthetizing the source of pain by injection, if the pain improves then the abnormality at the source was contributing for the pain. If on the other hand, the pain does not improve, then the abnormality was not the source of pain.

Types of Diagnostic Injections in the Spine

1. *Selective nerve root injection:* This helps block one of the major nerves coming out from the spine. This is diagnostically more superior than the epidural block.
2. *Medial branch block (MBB):* This helps determine whether the facet joints are the cause of pain when X-ray and scans are inconclusive in determining the source of pain. The facet joints are supplied by the medial nerves. If the pain disappears on injection then the facet joints are the source of pain and if the pain does not

improve, then the pain is not due to facet joint problems. The importance of this technique is that it helps perform a neurotomy if the facet joint in question is the source of pain. This will give an effective pain relief for six to eighteen months.

3. *Sacroiliac injection:* This helps to know if the Sacro-iliac joint is the source of pain. Discussed next.
4. *Discography:* This is also known as discogram. It helps us know that an abnormal looking MRI scan is the source of pain. If a normal disc is injected, there is no pain but if an abnormal disc is injected, it causes pain. After discography if the pain increases and resembles the pain patient is experiencing daily, then the test is said to be positive. However it has fallen into disrepute in modern days as it is not a very reliable diagnostic method and has its own limitations and drawbacks.

Therapeutic Injections

Injections are called therapeutic, when they relieve pain for more than the duration of the local anesthetics. These are also referred to as blocks. These may reduce the pain for weeks or months when successful. These injections only help to control the pain but will not cure a spine problem. The well known therapeutic spine injections are:

- Lumbar facet joint injection
- Epidural joint injection
- Medial branch neurotomy
- Sacro-iliac joint injection.

Now let us try to know in detail the lumbar facet joint injection and the epidural injections into the spine. The sacroiliac injection is dealt with separately.

Lumbar Facet Joint Injection

The facet joints are paired articular surfaces that are placed between the posterior aspects of two adjacent vertebrae. Flexion and rotation movements takes place in these joints. Facet nerve injection can be done by placing a spinal needle at the point where the superior articular surface and the transverse processes joint. Here the median branch passes over the cephalad edge of the transverse process.

Causes

- Flexion and extension injuries of the back
- Degenerative conditions like osteoarthritis.

Predisposing Factors

- Unaccustomed physical activity
- Poor posture
- Old injuries
- Poor nutritional status
- Psychological or behavioral abnormalities.

Presentation

- Pain in the affected joints.
- Spine movements are restricted and painful.

Signs

- On palpation tenderness could be elicited over the facet joints.

Methods

Two methods are described:

1. *Interarticular*: Here injection is given directly into the joint to block the pain.
2. *Nerve blocked*: Here the medial branch or the nerves that connect the joint are blocked. This helps determine whether the joint is indeed the source of pain.

Procedures

Position

- Prone with pillow under the anterior superior iliac spine to flatten the normal lumbar lordosis
- Drugs: 10 ml of 1 per cent lidocaine and 40 mg of methylprednisolone or 25 mg of triamcinolone
- Syringe: 2 ml and 10 ml/1 ½ inches/ 25-gauge needle/ 22 G spinal needle,end opening/non-ionic radio-opaque contrast medium
- Special equipments required are: C-arm, monitors, resuscitation equipments and drugs.

Techniques

- In the position mentioned above, the lumbar midline and an area of 10 by 5 cm on the lateral side is painted and draped

- Mark the spinous process of the vertebrae
- Identify the facet joint 2 to 3 cm lateral to the cephalic end of the spinous vertebrae by careful palpation
- Position the C-arm tilted 30 degrees to the sides of the joint to be injected and adjust the angle till the facet joint is clearly visualised
- Identify the point of insertion with the help of C-arm
- Infiltrate the skin at the point of insertion with 1 per cent lignocaine by raising a wheal
- Insert the spinal needle in a vertical direction to the skin till it enters the facet joint
- Do an aspiration test. If it is negative, then inject 0.5 ml of non-ionic radio-opaque contrast media. This will confirm the correct placement of the needle in the antero-posterior and oblique views
- After confirming the correct placement of the needle, inject a mixture of about 0.5 ml to 1 ml of the lignocaine and 40 mg of methylprednisolone or 25 mg of triamcinolone solution into the joint
- Inject the contents of the syringe gently.

Note: Do you know how to confirm a successful facet joint injection? Well it is the relief of pain.

Caution: Not more than 1 ml of total volume should be injected into a facet joint as it may damage it.

Resistance vs Inference

- If there is limited resistance; congratulations, you have hit the right spot

- If there is significant resistance; sorry, you are in the wrong space. Withdraw the needle, redirect and inject.

After care: At the injection site, after the injection

- Apply icepacks
- Apply a firm sterile bandage under pressure.

Complications

- Infection (hence follow strict aseptic measures)
- Transient increase of pain (seen in 25% of the cases)
- Ecchymosis
- Haematoma formation.

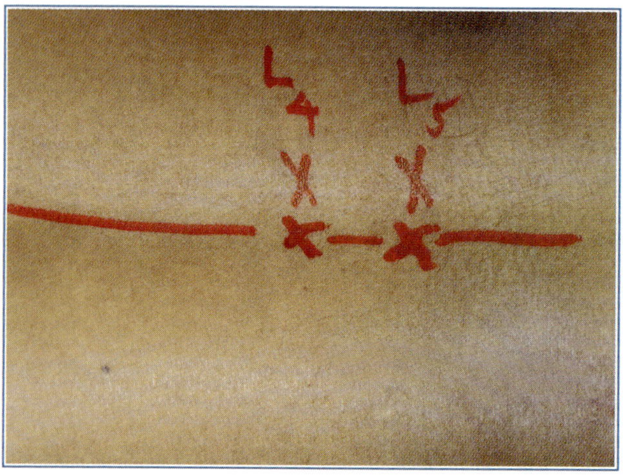

Fig. 3.8A: Mark the spinous process of the affected vertebra. Identify the facet joint 2-3 cm lateral to it

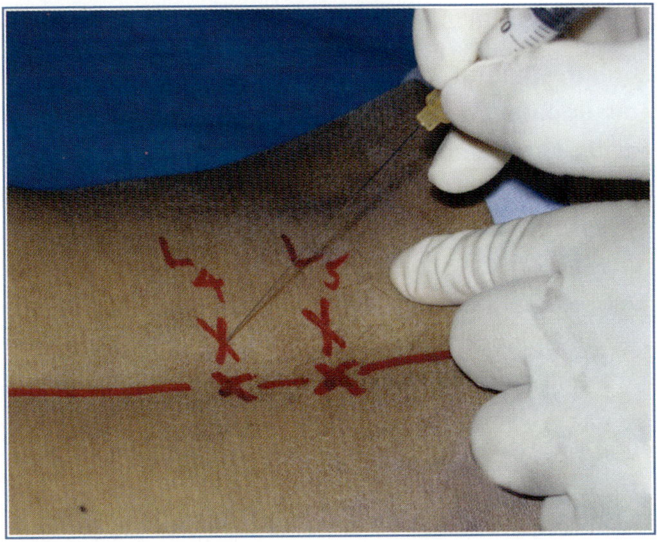

Fig. 3.8B: Insert the needle in a vertical direction to the skin till it enters the facet joint. Inject the contents after confirming the correct space with C-arm

Note: The incidence of ecchymosis and haematoma formation can be reduced if immediately after the injection, a firm sterile pressure bandage is applied.

Vital facts: Strictly observe the following after the injection:

- Simple analgesics and NSAIDs are advised
- To prevent the exacerbation of pain, avoid heat and gentle range of motion exercises for few days
- Avoid vigorous exercises for few days to prevent increase in pain.

Lumbar Epidural Injection

Lumbar epidural injection is indicated in lumbosacral radiculopathy wherein there is pain in the back and radiating pain along the buttock, posterior thigh and legs called the sciatica due to the compression of the affected nerve root usually the L5 and S1 nerve roots. The compression is usually due to herniated or prolapsed intervertebral disc due to prolonged intervertebral disc disease. Epidural space is the space inbetween the dura mater and the bony spinal canal.

Predisposing Factors

- Unaccustomed physical activity
- Poor posture
- Old injuries
- Poor nutritional status
- Psychological or behavioral abnormalities.

Presentation

- Pain in the back
- Sciatica
- Motor, sensory and reflex changes in the affected nerve root
- Spine movements are restricted and painful
- In sever disc prolapse there could be bladder and bowel changes.

Different Methods of Lumbar ESI

1. *Caudal block:* Here injection is given through sacral gap. Here the drugs are placed near the cauda equina and the chances of puncturing the dura are less.
2. *Translumbar:* This is the most common procedure. Here the needle is inserted between the spinous process of two vertebrae.
3. Transforaminal: This is a very selective injection given at the exit of a nerve root near its foramen. It has a diagnostic role and is commonly used in the neck.

Procedure of Translumbar Method

- Position: Lateral, usually lying on the side of the radiculopathy with the shoulder and buttocks parallel to the edge of the bed, perpendicular to the floor. The spine should be kept in a flexed position
- Drugs: 10 ml of 1 per cent lidocaine and 40 mg of methylprednisolone or 50 mg of triamcinolone/saline 10 ml
- Syringe: 2 ml and 10 ml/1 ½ inches/ 18, 20 and 22-gauge needle/18 G epidural set
- Special equipments required are: C-arm (optional), monitors, Resuscitation equipments and drugs.

Techniques

- In the position mentioned above, the lumbar midline and an area of 10 by 5 cm on the lateral side is painted and draped

- One per cent of 2 ml of lignocaine is drawn up into three 2 ml syringes
- One per cent of 2 ml of lignocaine and 50 mg of corticosteroid is drawn in a 10 ml syringe
- 10 ml of saline is drawn in another 10 ml syringe
- Identify the L 4-5 disc space which is situated on the intercrestal line by palpating the iliac crest on either side
- Palpate the spinous process of the affected vertebra and determine the level requiring the injection
- Confirm this by fluoroscopy.

Midline Approach

- Keep the index and the middle fingers of the left hand on either side of the interspace till the procedure of injection is completed
- With the right hand, Infiltrate the skin at the point of insertion with 1 per cent 2 ml lignocaine by raising a wheal
- Insert the epidural needle with its bevel facing the side of the radiculopathy in a direction of 60 degrees cephalad inbetween the index and middle fingers of the left hand, parallel to the floor, perpendicular to the spine, till the needle is gripped by the interspinous ligament
- With the left wrist leaning against the back of the patient, grip the hub of the needle with the index and middle fingers of the left hand and steady the needle
- Remove the stylet and apply the loss of resistance syringe containing normal saline

- Now advance the needle slowly and very carefully by applying constant pressure over the plunger
- The moment needle enters the ligamentum flavum, absolute resistance to the injection will be felt
- At this juncture, the needle is advanced very slowly till there is a sudden loss of resistance. This indicates the entry into the epidural space.
- Do an aspiration test for blood or CSF. If it is negative, then inject 3 ml of 1 per cent lignocaine
- Question the patient about the reduction of pain, or sensation or power in the lower limbs after 5 minutes
- If the procedure is being done for diagnostic purposes, the needle may be removed at this point and the procedure could be terminated

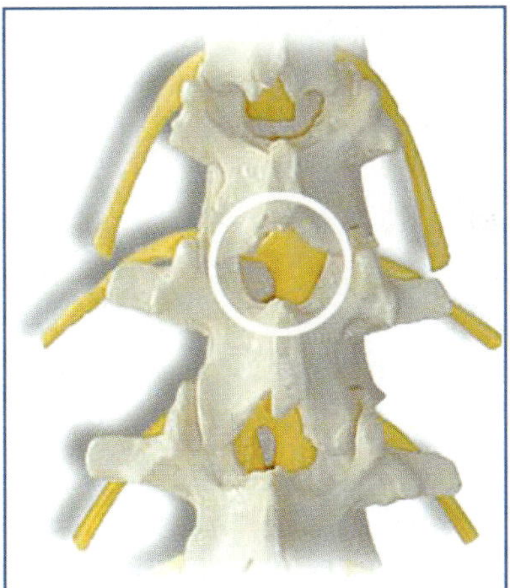

Fig. 3.9A: The interspinous space is the point of entry

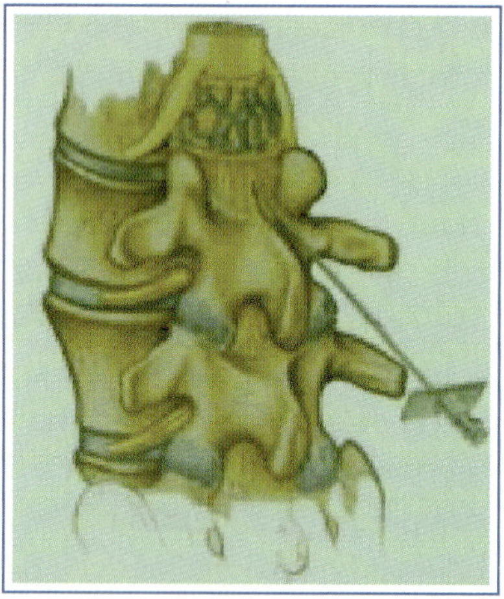

Fig. 3.9B: The translumbar method of epidural injection

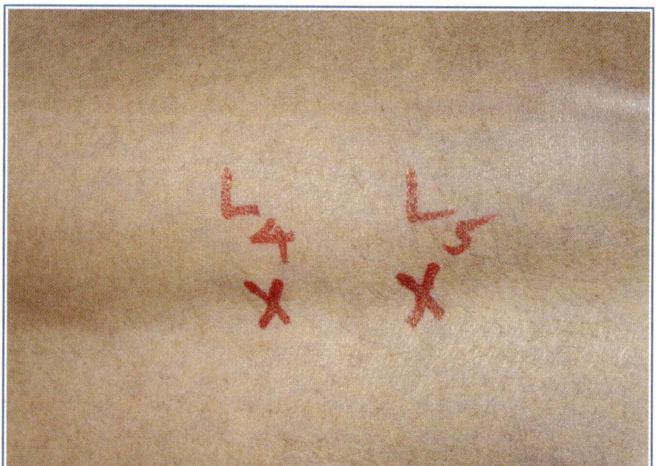

Fig. 3.9C: Mark the L_4 and L_5 spinous process with a sterile marker

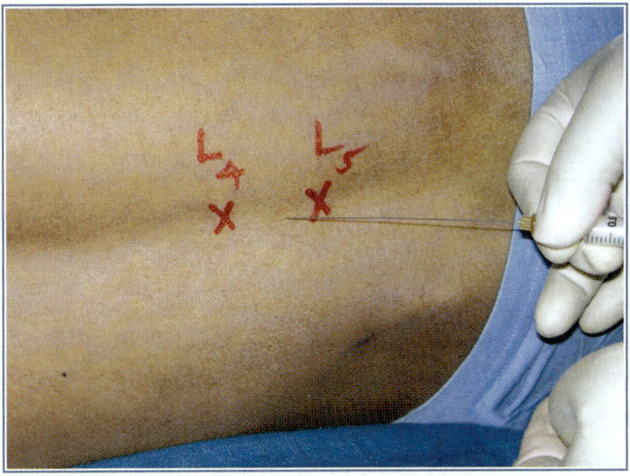

Fig. 3.9D: Epidural injection being given in the L_{4-5} disc space

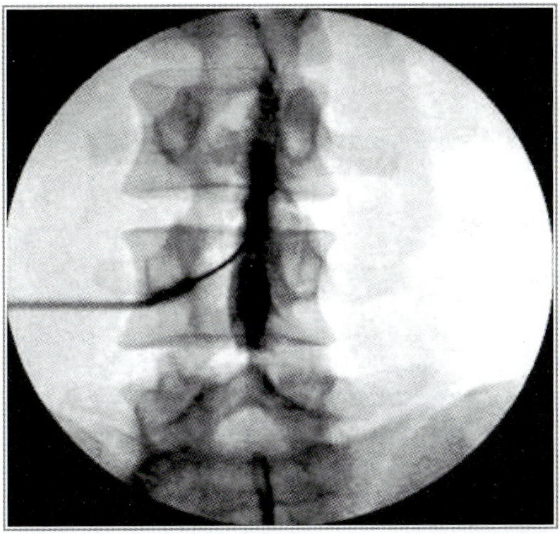

Fig. 3.9E: Confirmation of the placement of the needle into the epidural space by fluoroscopy

- But for therapeutic purposes a mixture of 2 ml of 1 per cent lignocaine and 50 mg of triamcinolone may be injected. Alternatively if indicated a catheter may be inserted through the needle
- Instruct the patient to lie on the side of pain in the lateral position for some time.

Do you know how to confirm a successful facet joint injection?
- Well it is the relief of pain
- By the anaesthesia in the distribution of the blocked nerve
- Improvement in straight leg raising test.

Note:
- *Air may be used instead of NACL*
- *An epidural catheter may be inserted through the needle and then the needle could be removed. However before injecting the drugs through the catheter, a test dose of lignocaine with or without adrenaline should be given*
- *A radio-opaque dye could be use to confirm the placement of the needle.*

Complications

Immediate

- Allergic reaction
- Failure to locate epidural space (then try with the sitting position)
- Injection into the blood vessels
- Intrathecal injection (test dose is important)
- Hypotension
- Headache.

Delayed

- Epidural abscess or bacterial meningitis due to infection
- Due to intrathecal injection there could be aseptic meningitis (hence test dose is important)
- Due to repeated steroid injections there could be cushingoid features.

Vital facts: Do you know in order the structures pierced to reach the epidural space? Mnemonic SILE:

- Supraspinous ligament
- Interspinous ligament
- Ligamentum flaxum
- Epidural space.

Section 4

Injection Techniques in the Lower Limbs

HIP AND PELVIS COMPLEX

INTRA-ARTICULAR INJECTION

The Hip Joint

Commonest indication for intra-articular injection into the hip joint is arthritis.

Causes for Arthritis

- Osteoarthritis—commonest cause
- Rheumatoid arthritis
- Post-traumatic arthritis.

Less Common

- Septic arthritis
- Lyme's disease
- Avascular necrosis
- Collagen vascular disease
- Villonodular synovitis.

Presentation

- Pain in the hip joint. It is localized around the hip and upper leg. Activity makes the pain worse
- Pain is constant and is dull aching
- Pain interferes with sleep
- Crepitus or popping sensation could be heard
- Gradual decrease in functional activity

- Decreased range of movements of the hip
- Simple day to day activities like walking, climbing stairs, squatting, getting in and out of the car, etc. are all affected.

Late Features

- Muscle wasting in and around the hip
- Frozen hip.

Procedures

- Position: Supine
- Drugs: 4 ml of 0.25 per cent preservative free bupivacaine and 40 mg of methylprednisolone
- Syringe: 2 ml/1 ½ inches/ 25-gauge needle
- Hip injection is usually carried out under fluoroscopy.

Techniques

- In the position mentioned above, the part is painted and draped
- Feel for the femoral pulse
- Identify the hip joint space which is two inches lateral and below the inguinal ligament
- Carefully insert the needle into the joint space
- If you hit the bone, withdraw the needle and redirect it more superiorly
- Inject the contents of the syringe gently.

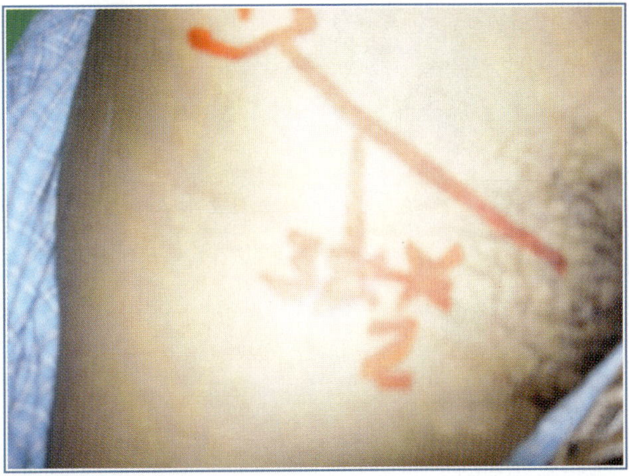

Fig. 4.1A: Identify the anterior superior iliac spine (Mark 1), and mark the inguinal ligament. Next feel for the femoral pulse (Mark 2) and mark a point two inches lateral to it (Mark 3)

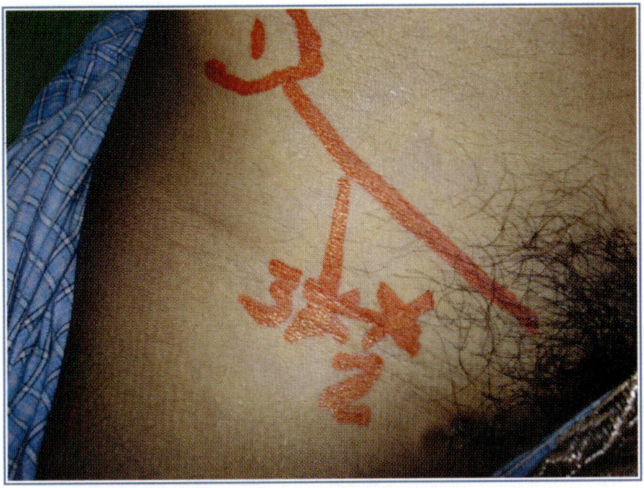

Fig. 4.1B: Mark 3 indicates the hip joint line

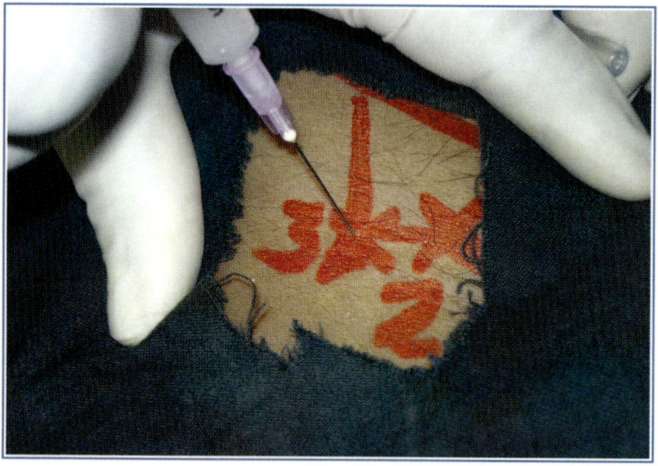

Fig. 4.1C: Carefully insert the needle vertically downwards into this point

Resistance vs Inference

- If there is limited resistance; congratulations, you have hit the right spot
- If there is significant resistance; sorry, you are in the wrong space. Withdraw the needle, redirect and inject.

After care: At the injection site, after the injection

- Apply icepacks
- Apply a firm sterile bandage under pressure.

Complications

- Infection (hence follow strict aseptic measures)
- Transient increase of pain (seen in 25% of the cases)

- Ecchymosis
- Haematoma formation.

Note: The incidence of ecchymosis and haematoma formation can be reduced if immediately after the injection, a firm sterile pressure bandage is applied.

Vital facts: Strictly observe the following after the injection:
- Simple analgesics and NSAIDs are advised
- To prevent the exacerbation of pain, avoid heat and gentle range of motion exercises for few days
- Avoid vigorous exercises for few days to prevent increase in pain.

The Sacroiliac Joint

Commonest indication for intra particular injection into the sacroiliac joint is arthritis.

Causes for Arthritis

- Osteoarthritis—commonest cause
- Rheumatoid arthritis
- Post-traumatic arthritis.

Less Common

- Ankylosing spondylitis
- Infection
- Lyme's disease
- Collagen vascular disease.

Rare Cause

Iatrogenically induced sacroiliact joint dysfunction due to overaggressive bone graft harvesting for spinal fusions.

Presentation

- Pain in the region of the sacroiliac joint. It is localized around the SI joint and upper thigh
- Pain radiates to the buttocks and upper thigh
- Pain does not radiate below the knee
- Activity makes the pain worse
- Pain is constant and is dull aching
- Pain interferes with sleep
- Rest and heat decreases the pain.

Clinical Findings

- Tenderness is present over the sacroiliac joint
- Spasm of the back muscles present
- Movements of the lumbosacral spine is reduced
- Pelvic compression test (pelvic rock test) is positive.

Investigations

- Laboratory tests
- Plain X-ray of the pelvis
- MRI.

Procedures

- Position: Prone
- Drugs: 4 ml of 0.25 per cent preservative free bupivacaine and 40 mg of methylprednisolone

- Syringe: 5 ml/3 ½ inches/ 25-gauge needle
- Usually requires a C-arm or CT-scan to confirm the placement of the needle.

Techniques

- In the position mentioned above, the point is painted and draped
- Palpate the posterior iliac superior spine and identify the SI joint space
- Carefully insert the needle into the joint space at an angle of 45 degrees under C-arm control
- If you hit the bone, withdraw the needle and redirect it more superiorly and laterally
- Inject the contents of the syringe gently.

Resistance vs Inference

- If there is limited resistance; congratulations, you have hit the right spot
- If there is significant resistance; sorry, you are in the wrong space. Withdraw the needle, redirect and inject.

After care: At the injection site, after the injection

- Apply icepacks
- Apply a firm sterile bandage under pressure.

Complications

- Infection (hence follow strict aseptic measures)
- Transient increase of pain (seen in 25% of the cases)
- Ecchymosis
- Haematoma formation.

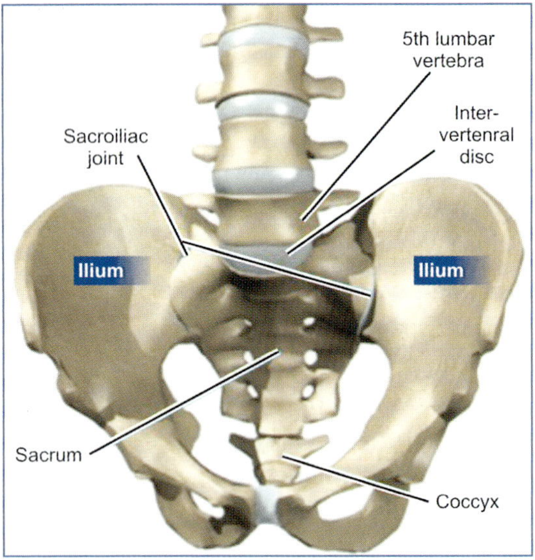

Fig. 4.2A: The bony anatomy of the pelvis and the SI joint

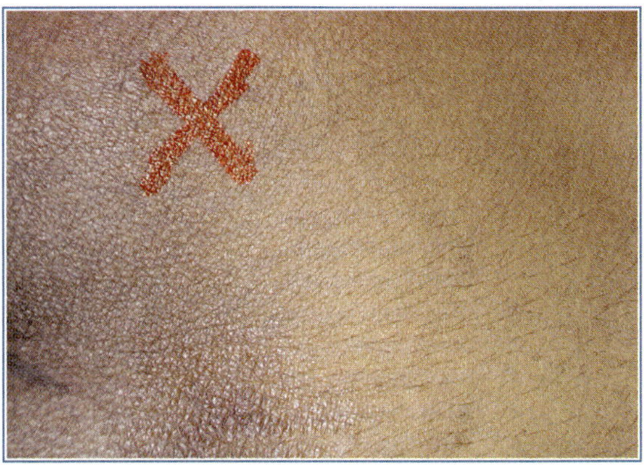

Fig. 4.2B: Palpate the posterior iliac spine and identify the SI joint space. Mark it with a sterile marker

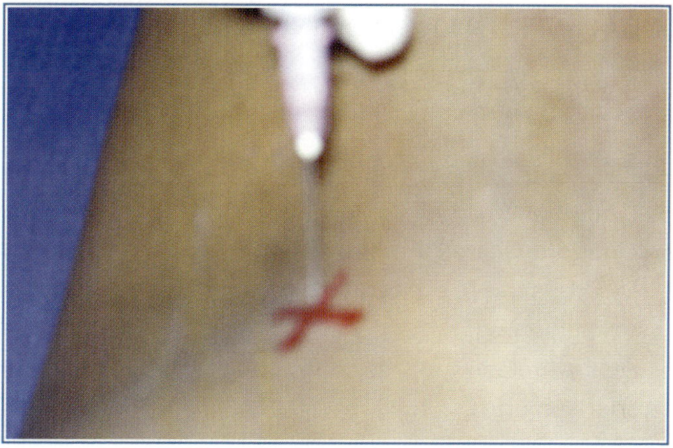

Fig. 4.2C: Insert the needle into the joint space at an angle of 45 degrees

Note: The incidence of ecchymosis and haematoma formation can be reduced if immediately after the injection, a firm sterile pressure bandage is applied.

Vital facts: Strictly observe the following after the injection:
- Simple analgesics and NSAIDs are advised
- To prevent the exacerbation of pain, avoid heat and gentle range of motion exercises for few days
- Avoid vigorous exercises for few days to prevent increase in pain.

LOCAL INFILTRATION OF INJECTION

Adductor Tendinitis

Causes

- Due to overuse
- Due to overstretch injuries
- Vigorous use of exercise equipment for lower extremity strengthening
- Acute stretching of the musculo-tendinous units as in sports injuries.

Presentation

- Pain in the region of the adductor tubercle
- Pain is sharp, constant and is severe
- Pain interferes with sleep
- Patient will demonstrate an adductor lurch type of gait (shifting the trunk over the affected extremity while walking)
- On palpation there is tenderness over the origin of the adductor tendons
- Pain increases on active resisted adduction and on passive abduction
- Gradual decrease in functional activity
- Decreased range of movements of the hip
- Simple day to day activities like walking, climbing stairs, squatting, getting in and out of the car, etc are all affected.

Late Features

- Muscle wasting in and around the hip
- Frozen hip.

Investigations

- Laboratory tests: This includes CBC, ESR, ANA, etc.
- Plain X-ray of the hip
- MRI scan is indicated if there is avascular necrosis or if there is a suspicion of an occult mass
- Injection technique is both diagnostic and therapeutic.

Procedures

- Position: Supine with the leg slightly adducted and externally rotated. This positioning allows access to the tendinous insertions of the hip adductor muscles
- Drugs: 2 ml of 0.25 per cent preservative free bupivacaine and 40 mg of methylprednisolone
- Syringe: 2 ml/1 ½ inches/ 25-gauge needle.

Techniques

- Patient is placed in the position mentioned above
- Identify the origin of the adductor tendons that lies 1½ inches lateral to the pubic symphysis from the pubic bone
- Prepare, paint and drape the area
- Carefully re-identify the point of origin of the adductor tendons

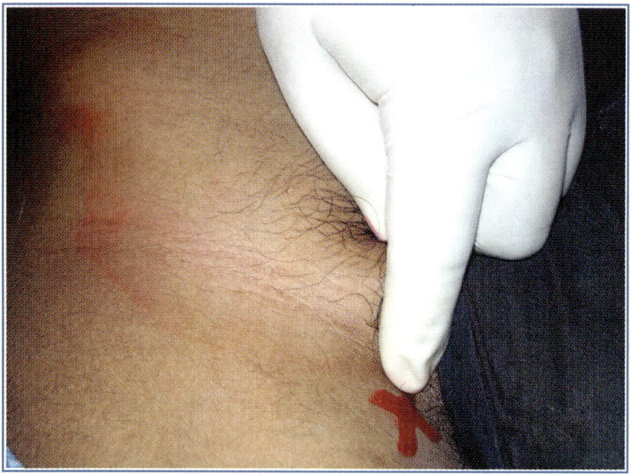

Fig. 4.3A: Identify the origin of the adductor tendon and mark it with a sterile marker

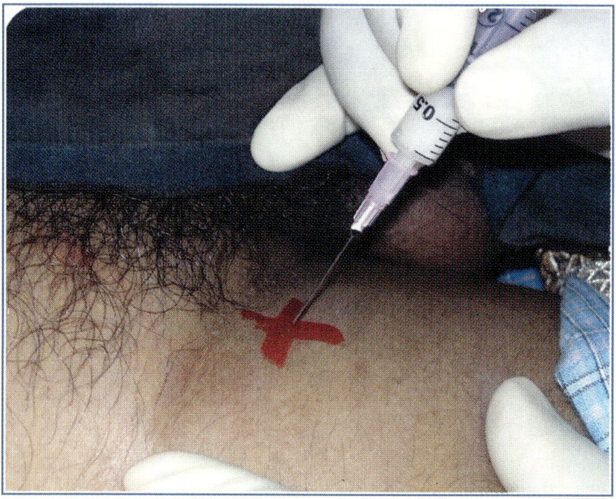

Fig. 4.3B: Insert the needle at this point perpendicular to the skin

- Carefully insert the needle perpendicular to the skin at this point till it touches the bone
- Withdraw the needle by 1 to 2 mm and Inject the contents of the syringe gently.

Resistance vs Inference

- If there is limited resistance; congratulations, you have hit the right spot
- If there is significant resistance; sorry, you are in the wrong space. Withdraw the needle, redirect and inject.

After care: At the injection site, after the injection

- Apply icepacks
- Apply a firm sterile bandage under pressure.

Complications

- Infection (hence follow strict aseptic measures)
- Transient increase of pain (seen in 25% of the cases)
- Rupture of the adductor tendons if they are directly injected
- Ecchymosis
- Haematoma formation.

Note: The incidence of ecchymosis and haematoma formation can be reduced if immediately after the injection, a firm sterile pressure bandage is applied.

Vital facts: Strictly observe the following after the injection:

- Simple analgesics and NSAIDs are advised
- To prevent the exacerbation of pain, avoid heat and gentle range of motion exercises for few days
- Avoid vigorous exercises for few days to prevent increase in pain.

Ischial Bursitis Pain

The ischial bursa lies between the ischial tuberosity and the gluteus maximus muscle. It may be single or multi-loculated.

Causes

- Acute trauma due to direct falls onto the buttocks
- Repeated micro-trauma due to overuse like prolonged riding of horses, bicycles, etc
- Running on irregular or soft surfaces.

Presentation

- Patient complains of pain at the base of the buttock and is brought about by resisted extension of the thigh
- Pain is localized over the ischial tuberosity and it could be referred to the hamstrings muscle on the affected side
- Patient is unable to sleep on the affected side
- Pain is sharp, catching especially when extending and flexing the hip on early morning first awakening
- Pain interferes with sleep
- There is point tenderness over the ischial tuberosity
- Passive straight leg raising test and active resisted extension of the affected leg reproduces the pain
- Sudden release of pressure during this procedure markedly increases the pain.

Investigations

- Laboratory tests: This includes CBC, ESR, ANA, etc.
- Plain X-ray of the hip
- MRI scan is indicated if rupture of the hamstrings muscles is suspected
- Injection technique is both diagnostic and therapeutic.

Procedures

- Position: Lateral with the affected side up and the affected leg flexed at the knee
- Drugs: 4 ml of 0.25 per cent preservative free bupivacaine and 40 mg of methylprednisolone
- Syringe: 5 ml/1 ½ inches/25-gauge needle.

Techniques

- Patient is placed in the position mentioned above
- Identify the ischial tuberosity with a gloved finger by deep palpation
- Prepare, paint and drape the area
- Carefully re-identify the ischial tuberosity
- Carefully insert the needle perpendicular to the skin at this point till it touches the bone
- Here the patient should experience paraesthesiae in the lower limb due to impingement of the needle on the sciatic nerve
- Now withdraw the needle and place it more medially
- Do a aspiration test
- If the aspiration test is negative and if there is no persistent paraesthesia, inject the contents of the syringe gently into the bursa.

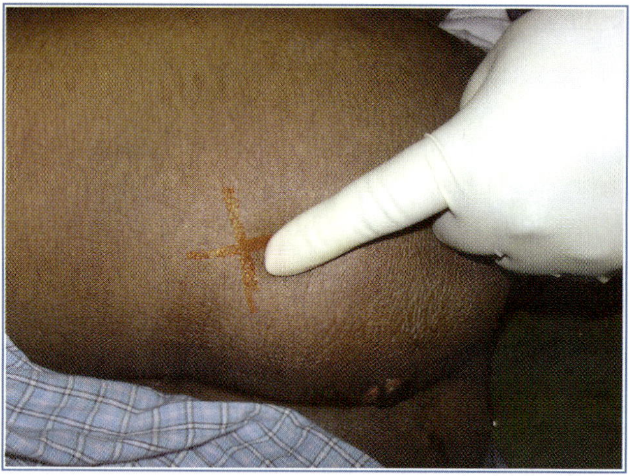

Fig. 4.4A: Identify the ischial tuberosity and mark it with a sterile marker

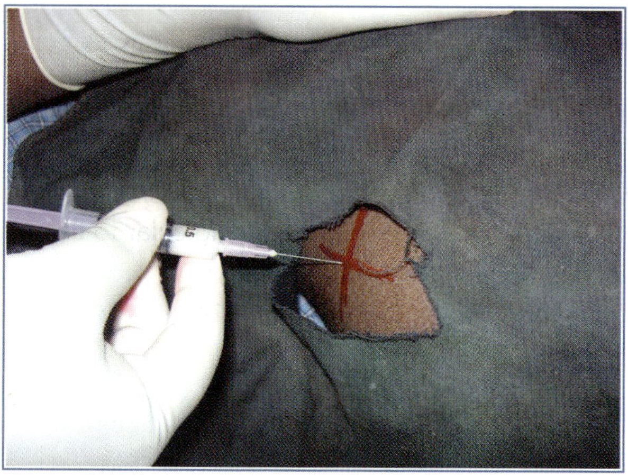

Fig. 4.4B: Insert the needle perpendicular to the skin at the marked point

Resistance vs Inference

- If there is limited resistance; congratulations, you have hit the right spot
- If there is significant resistance; sorry, you are in the wrong space. Withdraw the needle, redirect and inject

After care: At the injection site, after the injection

- Apply icepacks
- Apply a firm sterile bandage under pressure

Complications

- Infection (hence follow strict aseptic measures)
- Transient increase of pain (seen in 25% of the cases)
- Injury to the sciatic nerve
- Ecchymosis
- Haematoma formation.

Note: The incidence of ecchymosis and haematoma formation can be reduced if immediately after the injection, a firm sterile pressure bandage is applied.

Vital facts: Strictly observe the following after the injection:

- Simple analgesics and NSAIDs are advised
- To prevent the exacerbation of pain, avoid heat and gentle range of motion exercises for few days
- Avoid vigorous exercises for few days to prevent increase in pain.

Gluteal Bursitis Pain

The gluteal bursae lies between the gluteal maximus, medius and minimus muscles as well as between these muscles and the underlying bones. These bursae may be uni or multiloculated.

Causes

- Acute trauma due to direct falls onto the buttocks
- Repeated micro-trauma due to overuse like prolonged riding of horses, bicycles, etc
- Running on irregular or soft surfaces
- Repeated intramuscular injections.

Presentation

- Pain in the upper outer region of the buttocks
- Pain may be referred into the region of the sciatic notch
- Pain is sharp, constant and is severe
- Pain interferes with sleep
- Patient is unable to sleep on the affected side
- There could be a sharp catching sensation when extending and abducting the hip especially on first awakening
- On palpation there is tenderness over the gluteal bursa
- Pain increases on active resisted abduction and extension of the lower extremity and by passive flexion and abduction
- Sudden release of resistance during the above procedure markedly increases the pain.

Investigations

- Laboratory tests: This includes CBC, ESR, ANA, etc.
- Plain X-ray of the hip may reveal calcification

- MRI scan is indicated if there is a suspicion of an occult mass or tumor of the hip
- Injection technique is both diagnostic and therapeutic.

Procedures

- Position: Lateral with the affected side up and the affected hip and leg flexed at the knee
- Drugs: 4 ml of 0.25 per cent preservative free bupivacaine and 40 mg of methylprednisolone
- Syringe: 5 ml/3 ½ inches/ 25-gauge needle.

Techniques

- Patient is placed in the position mentioned above
- Identify the point of maximum tenderness within the upper and outer quadrant of the buttocks
- Prepare, paint and drape the area
- Carefully re-identify the point of pain
- Carefully insert the needle perpendicular to the skin at this point till it touches the wing of the iliac bone
- If the patient experiences paraesthesia along the course of the sciatic nerve when the needle is inserted, immediately withdraw it and redirect it more medially
- Do an aspiration test
- On hitting the bone, withdraw the needle by 1 to 2 mm and inject the contents of the syringe gently if the aspiration test is negative or if there is persistent paraesthesia.

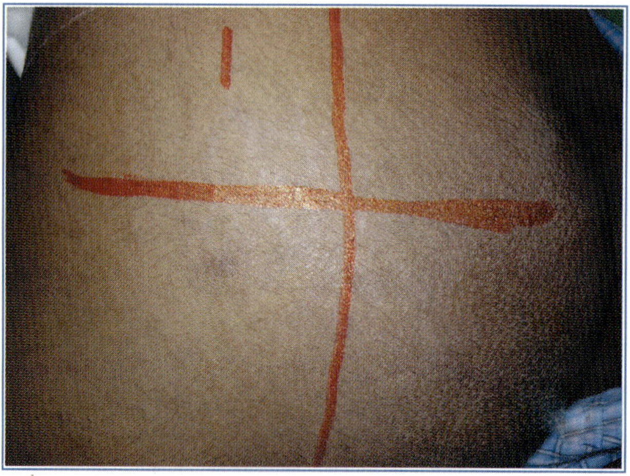

Fig. 4.5A: Divide the gluteal region into four quadrants. Mark the most tender point in the upper and outer quadrant

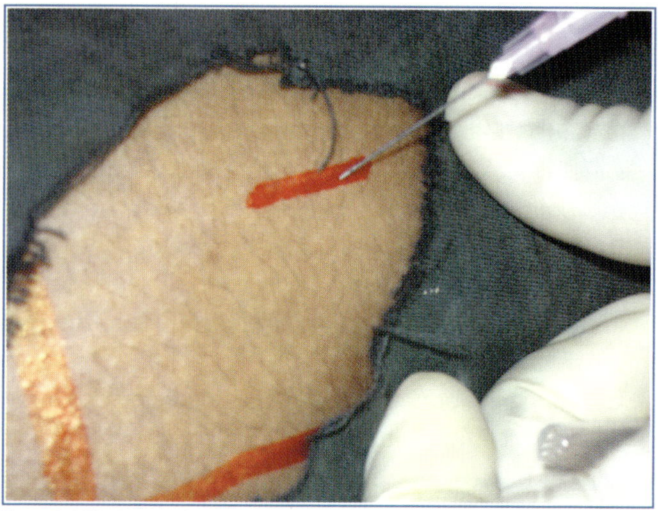

Fig. 4.5B: Insert the needle perpendicular to the skin at this point

Resistance vs Inference

- If there is limited resistance; congratulations, you have hit the right spot
- If there is significant resistance; sorry, you are in the wrong space. Withdraw the needle, redirect and inject.

After care: At the injection site, after the injection
- Apply icepacks
- Apply a firm sterile bandage under pressure.

Complications

- Infection (hence follow strict aseptic measures)
- Transient increase of pain (seen in 25% of the cases)
- Injury to the sciatic nerve
- Ecchymosis
- Haematoma formation.

Note: The incidence of ecchymosis and haematoma formation can be reduced if immediately after the injection, a firm sterile pressure bandage is applied.

Vital facts: Strictly observe the following after the injection:
- Simple analgesics and NSAIDs are advised
- To prevent the exacerbation of pain, avoid heat and gentle range of motion exercises for few days
- Avoid vigorous exercises for few days to prevent increase in pain.

Psoas Bursitis Pain

The psoas bursa lies medially in the femoral triangle between the anterior aspect of the neck of the femur and the psoas tendon in the femoral triangle. It may be uniloculated or multiloculated.

Causes

- Direct trauma to the psoas bursa due to seat belt injuries
- Due to overuse injuries from repeated flexion of the hip as in ballet dancers and javelin throwers.

Presentation

- Patient complains of pain in the groin
- Pain is localized to the area just below the crease of the groin anteriorly
- There could be referred pain into the hip joint
- Patient is unable to sleep on the affected side
- On movements of the hip there could be a sharp catching pain
- On palpation there could be point tendernss in the upper thigh just below the crease of the groin
- Passive flexion,adduction and abduction,active resisted flexion and adduction of the lower extremity causes pain
- Sudden release of resistance during the above procedure produces marked increase in the pain.

Investigations

- Laboratory tests: This includes CBC, ESR, ANA, etc.
- Plain X-ray of the hip may reveal calcification
- MRI scan is indicated if there is a suspicion of an occult mass or tumor of the hip
- Injection technique is both diagnostic and therapeutic.

Procedures

- Position: Supine
- Drugs: 9 ml of 0.25 per cent preservative free bupivacaine and 40 mg of methylprednisolone
- Syringe: 10 ml/3 ½ inches/ 25-gauge needle.

Techniques

- Patient is placed in the position mentioned above
- Identify the femoral pulse
- At a point 2 ½ inches down and lateral to the femoral artery pulsation, is the point of entry of the needle
- Prepare, paint and drape the area
- Carefully re-identify the point of pain
- Carefully Insert the needle at a 45 degrees angle medially and cephalad
- If the patient experiences paraesthesia along the course of the femoral nerve when the needle is inserted, immediately withdraw it and redirect it more laterally
- Do an aspiration test to rule out injury to the femoral vessels
- On hitting the bone, withdraw the needle by 1 to 2 mm and Inject the contents of the syringe gently if the aspiration test is negative or if there is persistent paraesthesia

Resistance vs Inference

- If there is limited resistance; congratulations, you have hit the right spot
- If there is significant resistance; sorry, you are in the wrong space. Withdraw the needle, redirect and inject.

After care: At the injection site, after the injection

- Apply icepacks
- Apply a firm sterile bandage under pressure.

Complications

- Infection (hence follow strict aseptic measures)
- Transient increase of pain (seen in 25% of the cases)
- Injury to the femoral nerve
- Injury to the femoral vesseels
- Ecchymosis
- Haematoma formation.

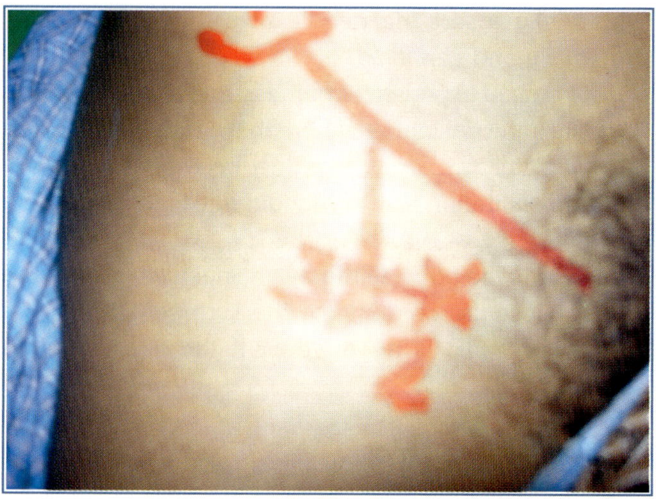

Fig. 4.6A: Identify the anterior superior iliac spine (Mark 1),and mark the inguinal ligament. Next feel for the femoral pulse (Mark 2) and mark a point two and a half inches lateral to it (Mark 3)

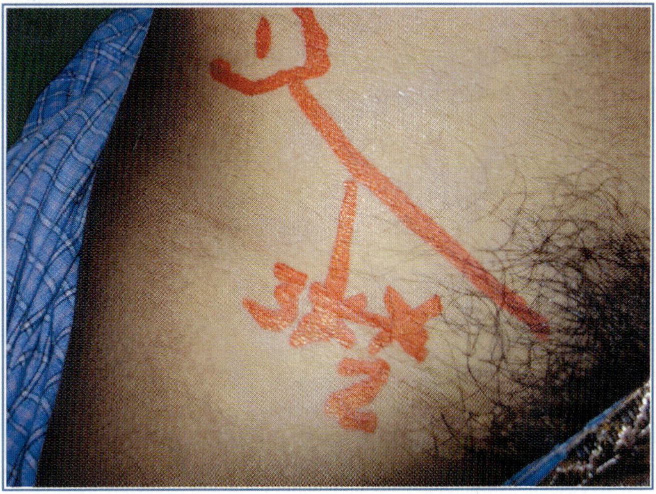

Fig. 4.6B: Mark 3 indicates the site of psoas abscess

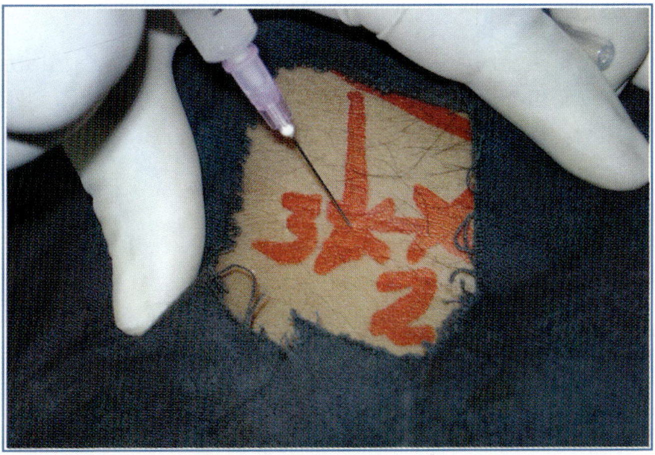

Fig. 4.6C: Carefully insert the needle at an angle of 45 degrees medially into this point

Note: The incidence of ecchymosis and haematoma formation can be reduced if immediately after the injection, a firm sterile pressure bandage is applied.

Vital facts: Strictly observe the following after the injection:
- Simple analgesics and NSAIDs are advised
- To prevent the exacerbation of pain, avoid heat and gentle range of motion exercises for few days
- Avoid vigorous exercises for few days to prevent increase in pain.

Trochanteric Bursitis Pain

The trochanteric bursa lies inbetween the greater trochanter and the tendon of the gluteus medius and the iliotibial tract. This bursa exists as a single locule or multiple locules.

Causes

- Acute trauma due to direct falls onto the greater trochanter
- Repeated micro-trauma due to running on irregular or soft surfaces
- Previous hip surgeries.

Presentation

- Pain in the lateral side of the hip
- Pain may radiate along the thigh and mimicks sciatica
- Pain is localized over the greater trochanter
- Pain is sharp, constant and is severe
- Pain interferes with sleep
- Walking upstairs is increasingly difficult

- Patient is unable to sleep on the affected side
- There could be a sharp catching sensation when the hip is moved especially on first awakening
- On palpation there is point tenderness over the lateral aspect of the upper thigh over the bursa
- Pain increases by passive adduction and abduction as well as active resisted abduction of the hip
- Sudden release of resistance during the above procedure markedly increases the pain.

Investigations

- Laboratory tests: This includes CBC, ESR, ANA, etc.
- Plain X-ray of the hip may reveal calcification
- MRI scan is indicated if there is a suspicion of an occult mass or tumor of the hip
- EMG helps differentiate from meralgia paresthetica and sciatica
- Injection technique is both diagnostic and therapeutic.

Procedures

- Position: Lateral with the affected side up and the affected hip and leg flexed at the knee at 30 to 50° and 60 to 90° respectively.
- Drugs: 2 ml of 0.25 per cent preservative free bupivacaine and 40 mg of methylprednisolone
- Syringe: 5 ml/3 ½ inches/ 25-gauge needle.

Techniques

- Patient is placed in the position mentioned above
- Identify the mid-point of the greater trochanter
- Prepare, paint and drape the area
- Carefully re-identify the point of pain
- Carefully insert the needle perpendicular to the skin at this point till it touches the greater trochanter
- If the patient experiences paraesthesia along the course of the sciatic nerve when the needle is inserted, immediately withdraw it and redirect it more laterally
- Do an aspiration test
- On hitting the bone, withdraw the needle by 1 to 2 mm and inject the contents of the syringe gently if the aspiration test is negative or if there is no persistent paraesthesia.

Resistance vs Inference

- If there is limited resistance; congratulations, you have hit the right spot
- If there is significant resistance; sorry, you are in the wrong space. Withdraw the needle, redirect and inject.

After care: At the injection site, after the injection

- Apply icepacks
- Apply a firm sterile bandage under pressure.

Complications

- Infection (hence follow strict aseptic measures)
- Transient increase of pain (seen in 25% of the cases)

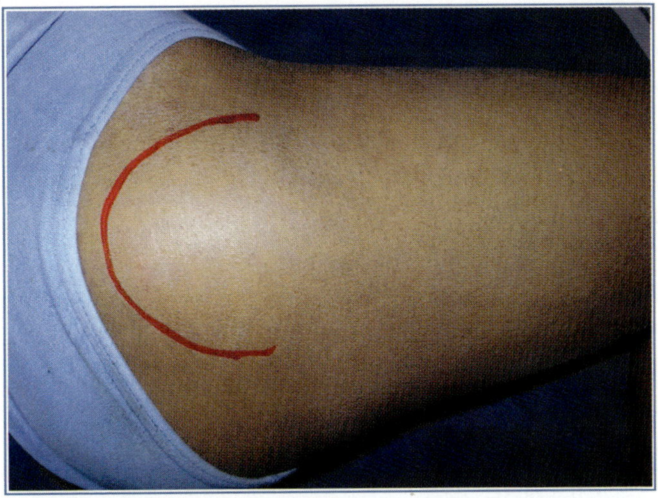

Fig. 4.7A: Identify and mark the greater trochanter

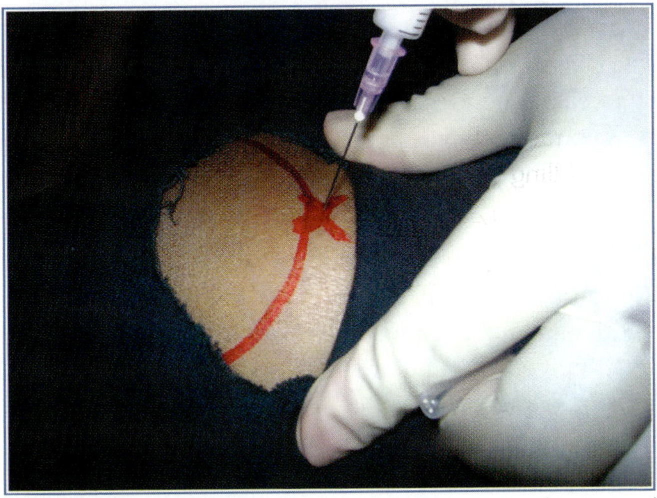

Fig. 4.7B: Identify the midpoint of the greater trochanter and insert the needle perpendicular to the skin till it touches the greater trochanter and inject

- Injury to the sciatic nerve
- Ecchymosis
- Haematoma formation.

Note: The incidence of ecchymosis and haematoma formation can be reduced if immediately after the injection, a firm sterile pressure bandage is applied.

Vital facts: Strictly observe the following after the injection:
- Simple analgesics and NSAIDs are advised
- To prevent the exacerbation of pain, avoid heat and gentle range of motion exercises for few days
- Avoid vigorous exercises for few days to prevent increase in pain.

MISCELLANEOUS

Osteitis Pubis Syndrome

This clinical syndrome is characterized by the following:
- Localized tenderness over the pubic symphysis
- Pain radiating into the inner thigh
- Waddling gait.

Causes

Common causes: It occurs most commonly following bladder, inguinal or prostate surgery. Infection spreads to the relatively avascular symphysis pubis through the hematogenous route.

Less Common Causes

- Rheumatoid arthritis
- Ankylosing spondylitis.

On Examination

- Point tenderness over the pubic symphysis
- On palpation over the pubic symphysis pain radiates to the inner thigh.
- Waddling gait in order to avoid movement of the pubic symphysis.

Note: The dysfunctional gait may cause lower limb bursitis and tendinitis.

Investigations

- Plain X-ray: Characteristic radiological changes seen are:
  - Erosion of the bony margins
  - Sclerosis
  - Widening of the symphysis pubis.
- Laboratory tests
- MRI SCAN to rule out occult tumor or mass
- Radio nucleotide bone scanning to rule out stress fractures
- Injection techniques are both diagnostic and therapeutic.

Procedures

- Position: Supine
- Drugs: 2 ml of 0.25 per cent preservative free bupivacaine and 40 mg of methylprednisolone
- Syringe: 2 ml/3 ½ inches/ 25-gauge needle.

Techniques

- In the position mentioned above, the point is painted and draped
- Identify *the midpoint of the pubic symphysis by careful palpation*
- Carefully insert the needle into the *center of the pubic symphysis at right angle to the skin till it touches the fibroelastic cartilage of the joint*
- Withdraw the needle slightly and do an aspiration for blood
- If aspiration test is negative and if there is no paraesthesiae, inject the contents of the syringe gently.

Resistance vs Inference

- If there is limited resistance; congratulations, you have hit the right spot
- If there is significant resistance; sorry, you are in the wrong space. Withdraw the needle, redirect and inject.

After care: At the injection site, after the injection

- Apply icepacks
- Apply a firm sterile bandage under pressure.

Complications

- Infection (hence follow strict aseptic measures)
- Transient increase of pain (seen in 25% of the cases)
- Ecchymosis
- Haematoma formation.

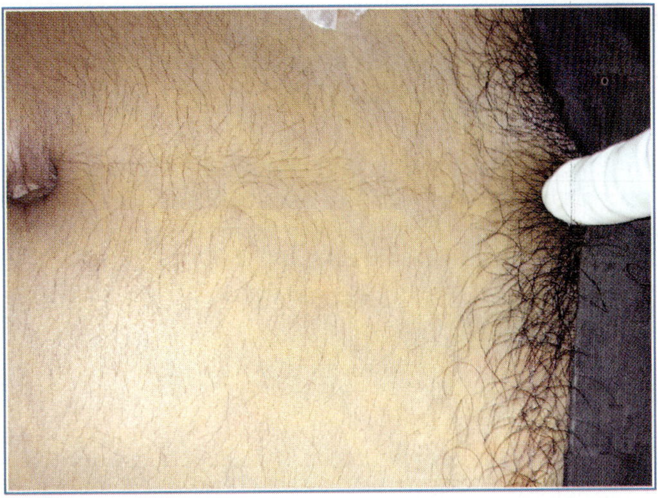

Fig. 4.8A: Identify the mid-point of the pubic symphysis

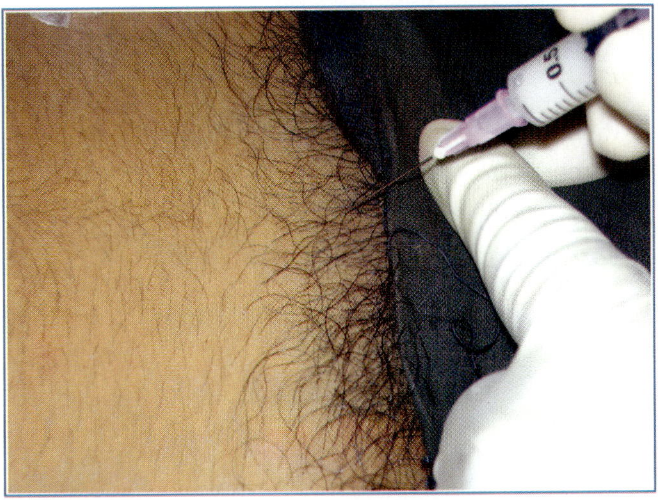

Fig. 4.8B: Insert the needle into the center of the pubic symphysis at right angles to the skin

Note: The incidence of ecchymosis and haematoma formation can be reduced if immediately after the injection, a firm sterile pressure bandage is applied.

Vital facts: Strictly observe the following after the injection:
- Simple analgesics and NSAIDs are advised
- To prevent the exacerbation of pain, avoid heat and gentle range of motion exercises for few days
- Avoid vigorous exercises for few days to prevent increase in pain.

Meralgia Paraesthetica

This is an entrapment neuropathy caused by compression of the lateral femoral cutaneous nerve by the inguinal ligament as it passes under or through that ligament.

Causes

- Trauma to the lateral femoral cutaneous nerve
- Compression over the nerve.

Presentation

- Pain and numbness, dysaesthesia in the upper lateral thigh
- Burning sensation in the same area
- These symptoms worsen on sitting, squatting, or wearing wide belts, etc.

Findings

- Tenderness is present over the lateral femoral cutaneous nerve at the anterior superior iliac spine and the inguinal ligament
- Tinel sign is positive
- Sensory deficit in the upper lateral thigh
- No motor deficit.

Differential Diagnosis

- Lumbar radiculopaty—lowbackache, reflex, motor and sensory change seen
- Diabetic femoral neuropathy
- Trochanteric bursitis
- Primary hip disorder.

Investigations

- Laboratory tests
- MRI SCAN to rule out occult tumor or mass
- Radionucleotide bone scanning to rule out stress fractures
- Injection techniques are both diagnostic and therapeutic.

Procedures

- Position: Supine position with pillow under the knees
- Drugs: 5-7 ml of 1 per cent preservative free bupivacaine and 40 mg of methylprednisolone
- Syringe: 10 ml/1 ½ inches/ 25-gauge needle.

Techniques

- In the position mentioned above, the point is painted and draped
- Identify the anterior superior iliac spine by careful palpation
- Mark a point one inch medial and inferior to the anterior superior iliac spine and the inguinal ligament
- Carefully insert the needle through this point perpendicular to the skin
- A popping sensation should be heard as it pierces the fascia at the external oblique muscle
- Withdraw the needle slightly and do an aspiration for blood
- After piercing the fascia of the external oblique muscle the drug is injected in a fan like manner
- If aspiration test is negative and if there is no paraesthesiae, inject the contents of the syringe gently.

Resistance vs Inference

- If there is limited resistance; congratulations, you have hit the right spot
- If there is significant resistance; sorry, you are in the wrong space. Withdraw the needle, redirect and inject.

After care: At the injection site, after the injection
- Apply icepacks
- Apply a firm sterile bandage under pressure.

Complications

- Infection (hence follow strict aseptic measures)
- Transient increase of pain (seen in 25% of the cases)

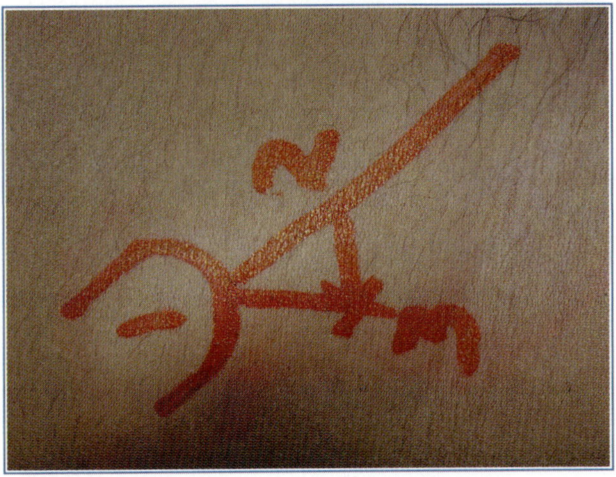

Fig. 4.9A: Identify the anterior superior iliac spine (Mark 1). Mark the inguinal ligament (Mark 2)

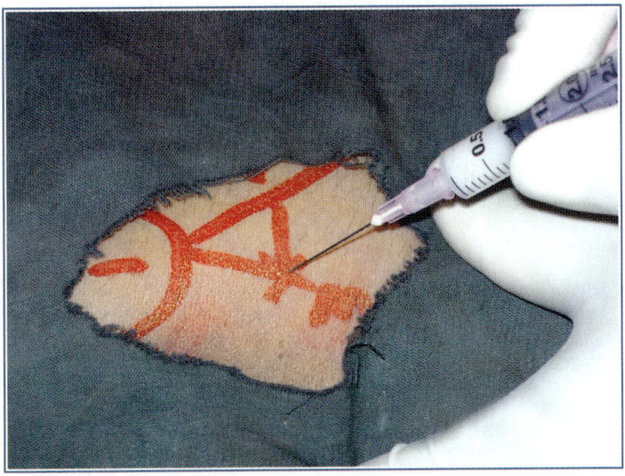

Fig. 4.9B: Mark a point one inch medial and inferior above two points. Insert the needle perpendicular to the skin at this point

- Ecchymosis
- Haematoma formation.

Note: The incidence of ecchymosis and haematoma formation can be reduced if immediately after the injection, a firm sterile pressure bandage is applied.

Vital facts: Strictly observe the following after the injection:
- Simple analgesics and NSAIDs are advised
- To prevent the exacerbation of pain, avoid heat and gentle range of motion exercises for few days
- Avoid vigorous exercises for few days to prevent increase in pain.

Complications

- Damage to the femoral vessels
- Damage to the peritoneal cavity and colon
- Infection
- Ecchymosis and haematoma.

Coccydynia Syndrome

It is a common pain syndrome that is characterized by pain localized to the tailbone that radiates to the lower sacrum and perineum. It is more commonly seen in females.

Causes

- Direct injury to the coccyx due to fall or kick
- May be seen after difficult vaginal delivery
- Strain of the sacrococcygeal ligament
- Fracture of the coccyx
- Arthritis of the sacrococcygeal joint.

Presentation

- Pain in the coccygeal region
- Difficulty in sitting, etc
- To avoid pressure on the coccyx patient sits on one buttock.

Findings

- Point tenderness over the coccyx
- Movements of the coccyx increases the pain
- Movements of the coccyx may cause sharp paraesthesiae into the rectum
- On per rectal examination there could be induration of the levator ani, piriformis and coccygeus muscles. Palpation induces severe spasm.

Investigations

- Laboratory tests
- Plain X-ray—to rule out occult bony pathology and tumor
- MRI scan to rule out occult tumor or mass
- Radio nucleotide bone scanning to rule out stress fractures
- Injection techniques are both diagnostic and therapeutic.

Procedures

- Position: Prone with the head placed on a pillow and turned away from the doctor. The legs and heels are abducted and the limbs are internally rotated. Note: The position prevents tightening of the gluteal muscles and enables to make identification of the sacrococcygeal joint easily

- Drugs: 5 ml of 1 per cent preservative free lidocaine and 40 mg of methylprednisolone
- Syringe: 10 ml/ 1½ inches/ 25-gauge needle.

Techniques

- In the position mentioned above, the point is painted and draped
- Place the middle finger of the non-dominant hand over the sterile drape into the natal cleft and at the base of the sacrum and palpate the sacrococcygeal joint with the fingertip
- Now carefully insert the needle at an angle of 45 degrees into the region of the sacrococcygeal ligament and joint
- If the ligament is successfully penetrated a pop will be felt and heard
- Withdraw the needle slightly and do an aspiration for blood or CSF
- If aspiration test is negative and if there is no paraesthesiae, inject the contents of the syringe gently.

Caution: If the aspiration test is positive for either, then abandon the procedure and do not attempt it within the next 24 hours.

Resistance vs Inference

- If there is limited resistance; congratulations, you have hit the right spot
- If there is significant resistance; sorry, you are in the wrong space. Withdraw the needle, redirect and inject.

After care: At the injection site, after the injection

- Apply icepacks
- Apply a firm sterile bandage under pressure.

Complications

- Infection (hence follow strict aseptic measures)
- Transient increase of pain (seen in 25% of the cases)
- Ecchymosis
- Haematoma formation.

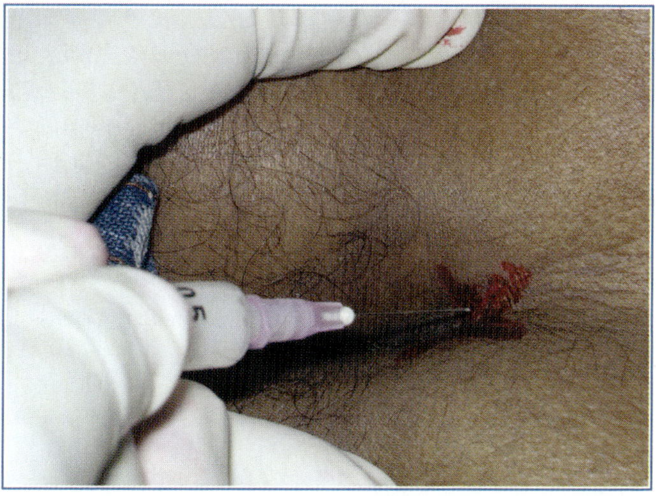

Fig. 4.10A: Palpate the sacrococcygeal joint and mark it with a sterile marker

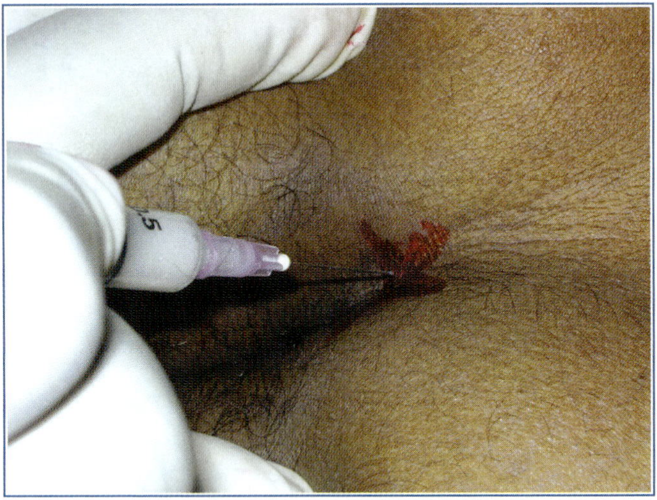

Fig. 4.10B: Insert the needle at an angle of 45 degrees into the marked point

Note: The incidence of ecchymosis and haematoma formation can be reduced if immediately after the injection, a firm sterile pressure bandage is applied.

Vital facts: Strictly observe the following after the injection:

- Simple analgesics and NSAIDs are advised
- To prevent the exacerbation of pain, avoid heat and gentle range of motion exercises for few days
- Avoid vigorous exercises for few days to prevent increase in pain.

KNEE JOINT COMPLEX

KNEE JOINT

Approaches to the Knee Joint

There are four major approaches to the knee:

1. *Medial retropatellar approach:* this approach is preferred in moderate or large effusion and this is the easiest. It consists of the following steps:
   - Patient is supine with the knee extended
   - The quadriceps muscles should be kept relaxed so that the patella is not clamped firmly on the femoral condyles. This will prevent the entry of the needle into the joint
   - The site of entry is just below the midpoint of the patella on the medial side
   - Introduce the needle towards the direction of the suprapatellar pouch
   - After about penetration for 1.5 cm the fluid may be aspirated
   - To prevent damage to the articular cartilage do not insert the needle deep
   - Milk the suprapatellar pouch as the fluid is being aspirated.
2. *Lateral retropatellar approach:* This consists of the following steps:
   - Patient is in the same position as mentioned above
   - The point of injection is the junction of the upper and middle thirds of the patella

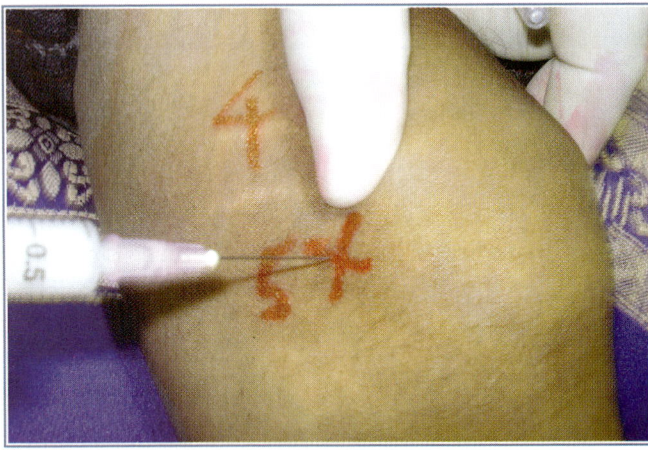

Fig. 4.11A: Medial midpatellar approach

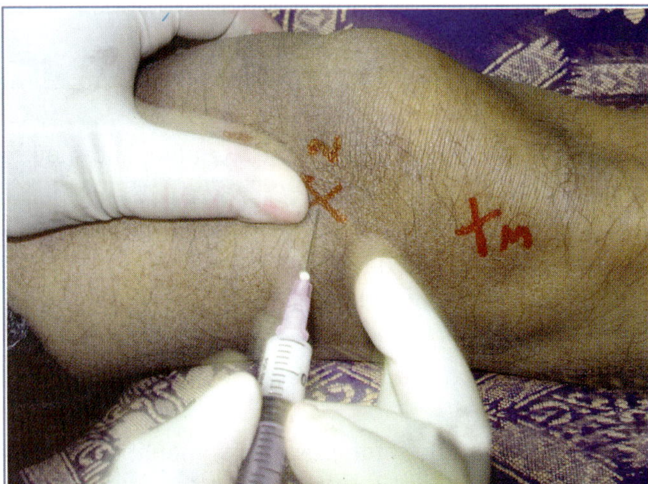

Fig. 4.11B: Lateral retropatellar approach

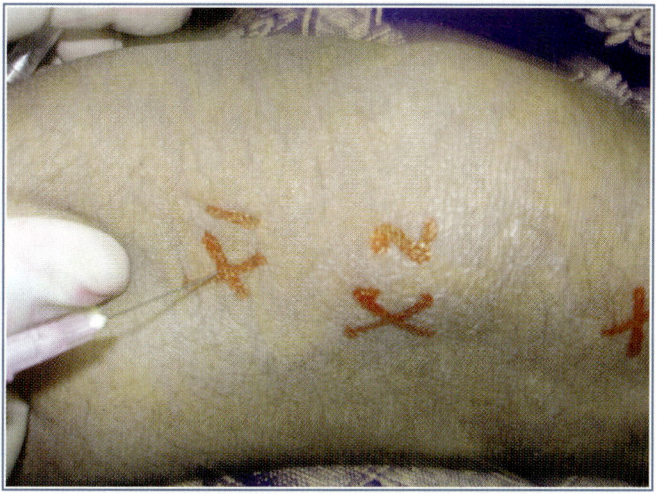

Fig. 4.11C: Superolateral approach

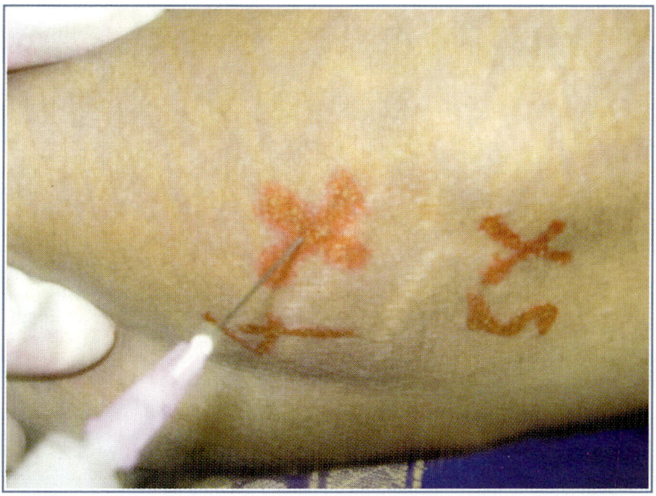

Fig. 4.11D: Superomedial approach

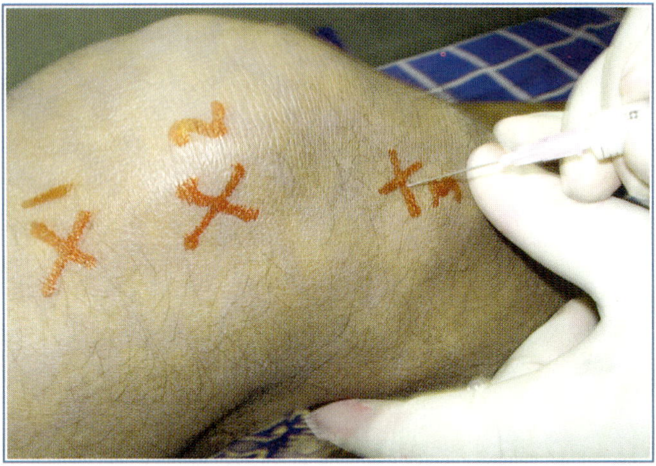

Fig. 4.11E: Infrapatellar lateral approach

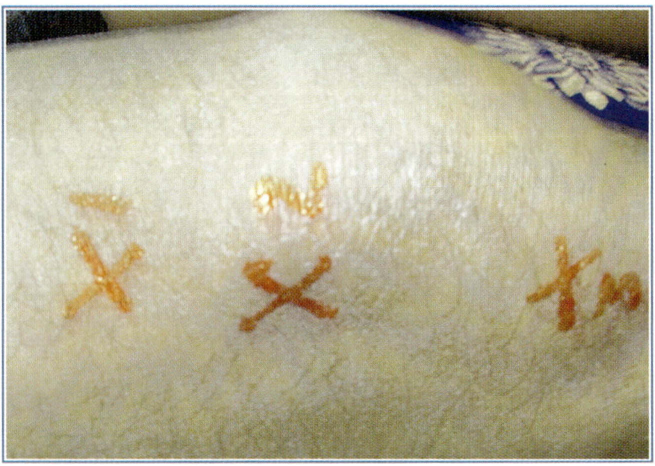

Fig. 4.11F: Various lateral approaches for the knee

- To increase the gap between the patella and femur laterally, push the patella out from the medial side
- Insert the needle in the point mentioned above in the direction of the suprapatellar pouch
- To prevent the needle from pushing it too far, keep aspirating as soon as the needle is introduced.

3. *Suprapatellar approach:* In very large effusions the suprapatellar pouch is expanded. The needle can be introduced directly into the pouch just lateral to the patella.
4. *Anterior approach:* This consists of the following steps:
   - The knee is flexed to 90 degrees
   - The needle is introduced just below the patella pole on to the side of the patellar tendon
   - The needle is introduced into the intercondylar fossa between the medial and lateral condyles after 4 to 5 cm parallel to the line of the tibial plateau
   - This approach avoids the risk of injury to the articular cartilage
   - However, it is rarely used nowadays.

INTRA-ARTICULAR INJECTION

Knee Joint Arthritis

Commonest indication for intra-articular injection into the knee joint is arthritis.

Causes for Arthritis

- Osteoarthritis—commonest cause
- Rheumatoid arthritis
- Post-traumatic arthritis.

Less Common

- Old septic arthritis
- Lyme's disease
- Collagen vascular disease
- Villonodular synovitis.

Presentation

- Pain in the knee joint. It is localized around the knee and upper leg
- Activity makes the pain worse
- Pain is constant and is dull aching
- Pain interferes with sleep
- Crepitus or popping sensation could be hard
- Gradual decrease in functional activity
- Decreased range of movements of the knee
- Simple day to day activities like walking, climbing stairs, squatting, getting in and out of the car, etc are all affected.

Late Features

- Muscle wasting in and around the knee
- Joint instability.

Investigations

- Laboratory tests
- Plain X-ray—to rule out occult bony pathology and tumor

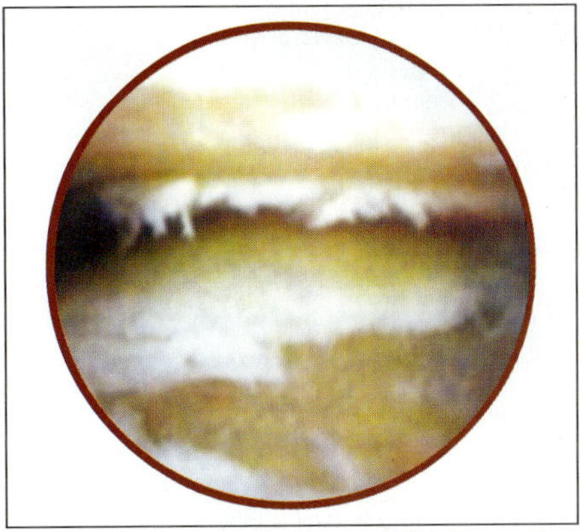

Fig. 4.12A: Arthroscopic view of OA knee showing degenerated cartilages

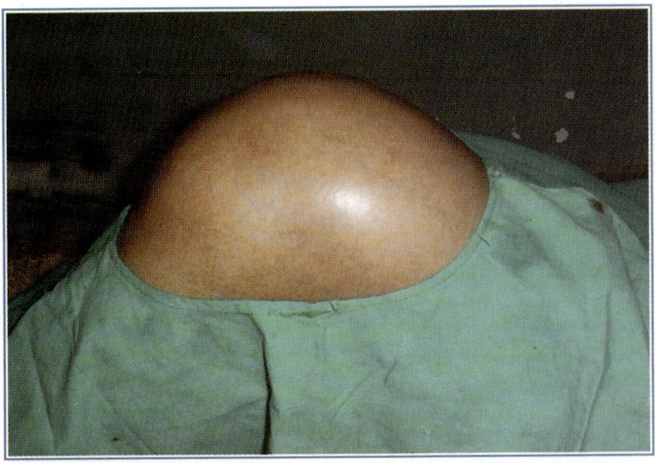

Fig. 4.12B: The knee is in flexion and is painted and draped

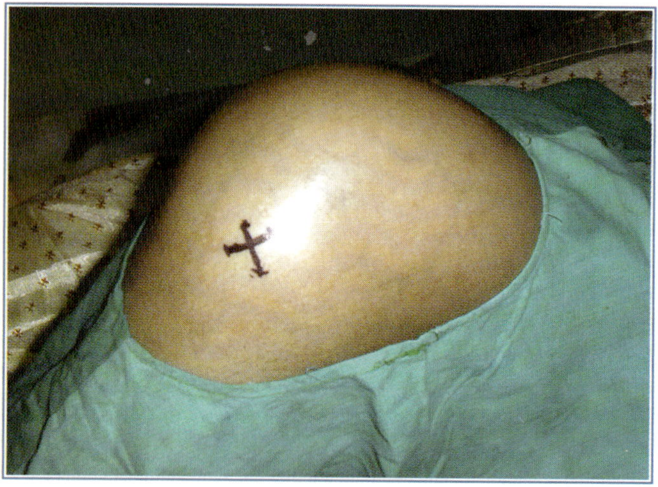

Fig. 4.12C: Identify the depression by the side of the ligamentum patella on the down and lateral side and mark it

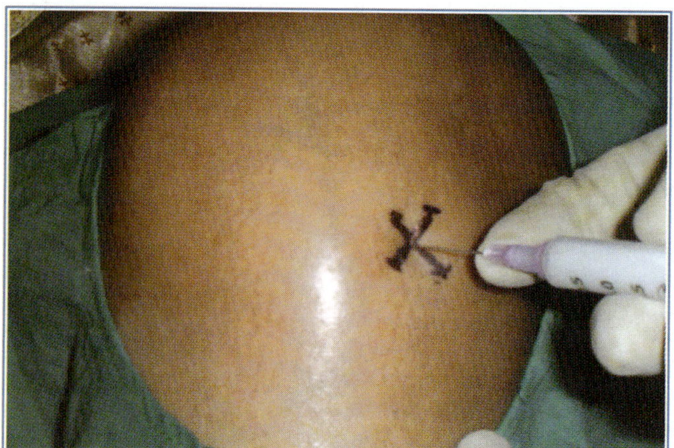

Fig. 4.12D

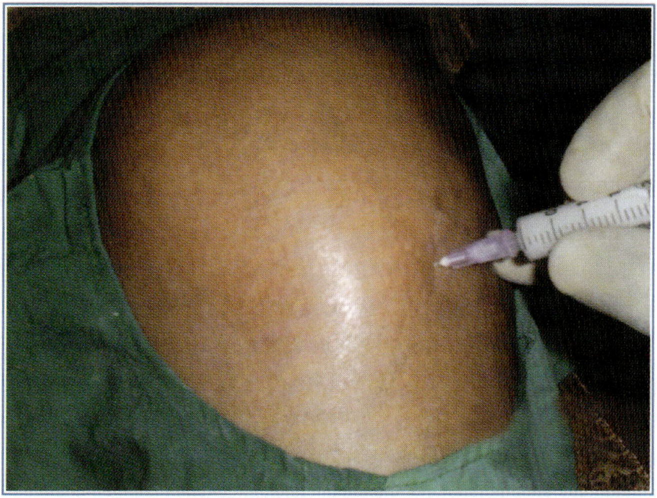

Fig. 4.12E

Figs 4.12D and E: Insert the needle into the joint at the marked site

- MRI scan
- Radionucleotide bone scanning to rule out stress fractures

Injection techniques are both diagnostic and therapeutic.

Procedures

- Position: Supine with knee flexed to varying degrees
- Drugs: 5 ml of 0.25 per cent preservative free bupivacaine and 40 mg of methylprednisolone
- Syringe: 5 ml/1 ½ inches/ 25-gauge needle.

Techniques

- In the position mentioned above, the part is painted and draped
- Push the patella to the medial side
- Identify the knee joint space which is felt as a depression between the femoral and tibial condyles
- Carefully insert the needle into the joint space in between the patella and the femoral condyles at the middle of the medial edge of the patella
- If you hit the bone, withdraw the needle and redirect it more superiorly
- Advance the needle carefully into the joint space
- Inject the contents of the syringe gently.

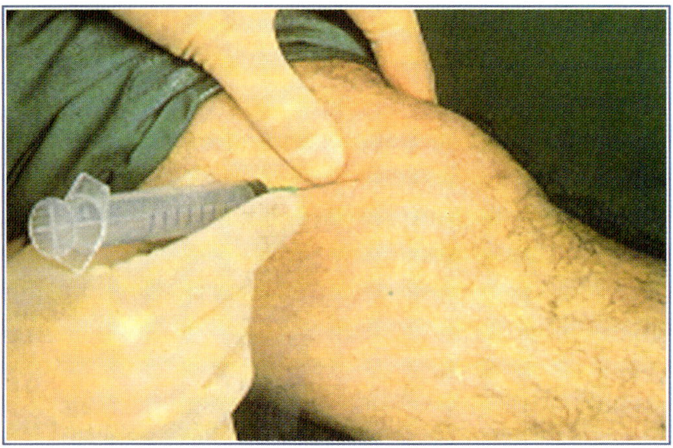

Fig. 4.13: Medial approach

Resistance vs Inference

- If there is limited resistance; congratulations, you have hit the right spot
- If there is significant resistance; sorry, you are in the wrong space. Withdraw the needle, redirect and inject.

After care: At the injection site, after the injection

- Apply icepacks
- Apply a firm sterile bandage under pressure.

Complications

- Infection (hence follow strict aseptic measures)
- Transient increase of pain (seen in 25% of the cases)
- Ecchymosis
- Haematoma formation.

Note: The incidence of ecchymosis and haematoma formation can be reduced if immediately after the injection, a firm sterile pressure bandage is applied.

Vital facts: Strictly observe the following after the injection:

- Simple analgesics and NSAIDs are advised
- To prevent the exacerbation of pain, avoid heat and gentle range of motion exercises for few days
- Avoid vigorous exercises for few days to prevent increase in pain.

LOCAL INFILTRATION FOR THE SOFT TISSUE LESIONS AROUND THE KNEE

Medial Collateral Ligament Sprain

It is due to trauma to the medial aspect of the knee from falls with the leg in valgus and externally rotated.

Site

The medial collateral ligament is usually susceptible to injury at the joint line or avulsion at its origin or insertion.

Presentation

- Pain over the medial joint line
- Pain increases on valgus and external rotation of the knee
- Activity increases the pain, rest relieves it
- Pain is constant and dull aching
- Pain may interfere with sleep.

Investigations

- Laboratory tests
- Plain X-ray—to rule out occult bony pathology and tumor
- MRI scan
- Radionucleotide bone scanning to rule out stress fractures
- Injection techniques are both diagnostic and therapeutic.

Procedures

- Position: Supine with knee slightly bent
- Drugs: 2 ml of 0.25 per cent preservative free bupivacaine and 40 mg of methylprednisolone
- Syringe: 2 ml/1 ½ inches/ 25-gauge needle.

Techniques

- In the position mentioned above, the part is painted and draped
- Identify the most tender portion of the ligament
- Carefully insert the needle at an angle of 45 degrees angle to the skin

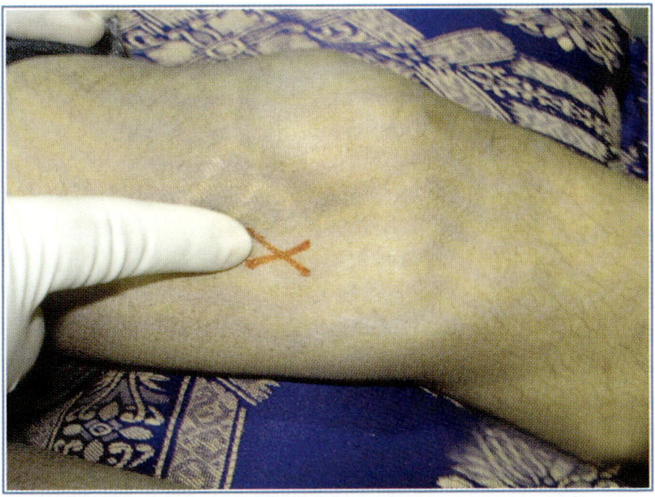

Fig. 4.14A: Identify the most tender point on the medial side of the knee joint and mark it with a sterile marker

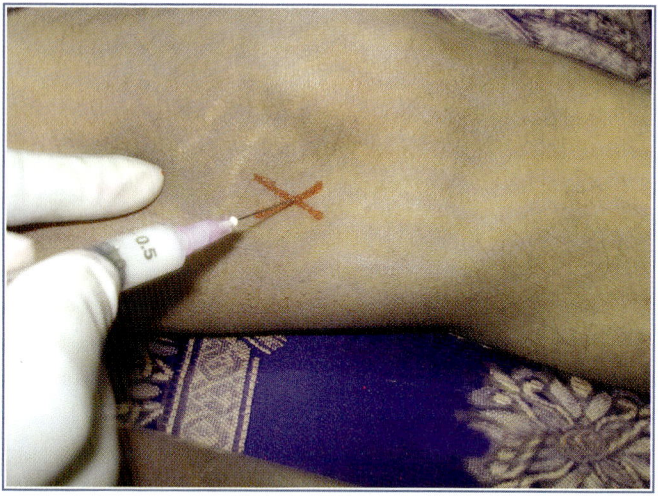

Fig. 4.14B: Insert the needle 45 degrees to the skin at this point

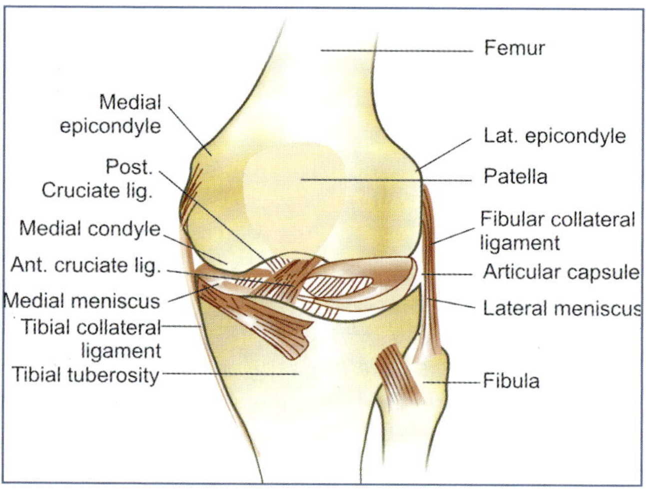

Fig. 4.14C: Shows the various ligaments of the knee joint

- If you hit the bone, withdraw the needle and redirect it more superiorly
- Inject the contents of the syringe gently.

Resistance vs Inference

- If there is limited resistance; congratulations, you have hit the right spot
- If there is significant resistance; sorry, you are in the wrong space. Withdraw the needle, redirect and inject.

After care: At the injection site, after the injection
- Apply icepacks
- Apply a firm sterile bandage under pressure.

Complications

- Infection (hence follow strict aseptic measures)
- Transient increase of pain (seen in 25% of the cases)
- Ecchymosis
- Haematoma formation.

Note: The incidence of ecchymosis and haematoma formation can be reduced if immediately after the injection, a firm sterile pressure bandage is applied.

Vital facts: Strictly observe the following after the injection:
- Simple analgesics and NSAIDs are advised
- To prevent the exacerbation of pain, avoid heat and gentle range of motion exercises for few days
- Avoid vigorous exercises for few days to prevent increase in pain.

Quadriceps Expansion Syndrome

It is characterized by pain at superior pole of the patella mainly on the medial side.

Causes

- Overuse of the knee
- Misuse of the knee
- Direct trauma to the quadriceps tendon
- Acute calcific tendinits due to acute strain injuries.

Presentation

- Pain over the superomedial aspect of the knee.
- Activity increases the pain
- It increases on walking down slopes or stairs
- It interferes with sleep
- Active resisted extension of the knee reproduces the pain
- Tenderness over the superomedial edge of the patella.

Investigations

- Laboratory tests
- Plain X-ray—to rule out occult bony pathology and tumor
- MRI scan
- Radionucleotide bone scanning to rule out stress fractures
- Injection techniques are both diagnostic and therapeutic.

Procedures

- Position: Supine with knee slightly flexed by a small pillow
- Drugs: 2 ml of 0.25 per cent preservative free bupivacaine and 40 mg of methylprednisolone
- Syringe: 5 ml/1 ½ inches/ 25-gauge needle.

Techniques

- In the position mentioned above, the part is painted and draped
- Identify the medial edge of the superior pole of the patella.
- Carefully Insert the needle horizontally towards the medial edge of the patella until it impinges on the bone
- Now slightly withdraw the needle
- Inject the contents of the syringe gently.

Resistance vs Inference

- If there is limited resistance; congratulations, you have hit the right spot
- If there is significant resistance; sorry, you are in the wrong space. Withdraw the needle, redirect and inject.

After care: At the injection site, after the injection

- Apply icepacks
- Apply a firm sterile bandage under pressure.

Complications

- Infection (hence follow strict aseptic measures)
- Transient increase of pain (seen in 25% of the cases)

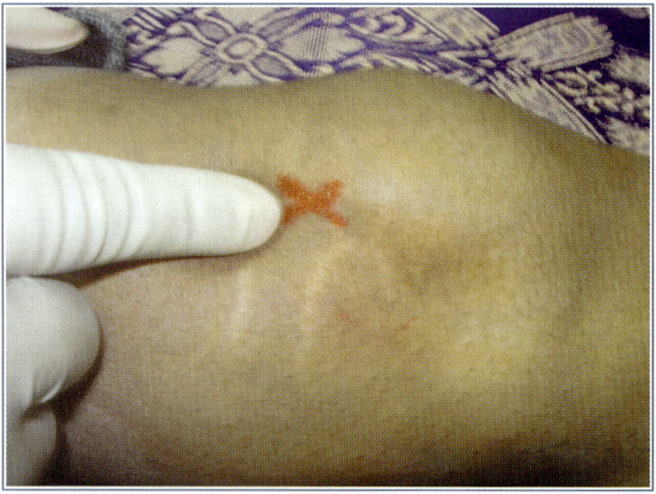

Fig. 4.15A: Identify the medial edge of the superior pole of the patella and mark it with a sterile marker

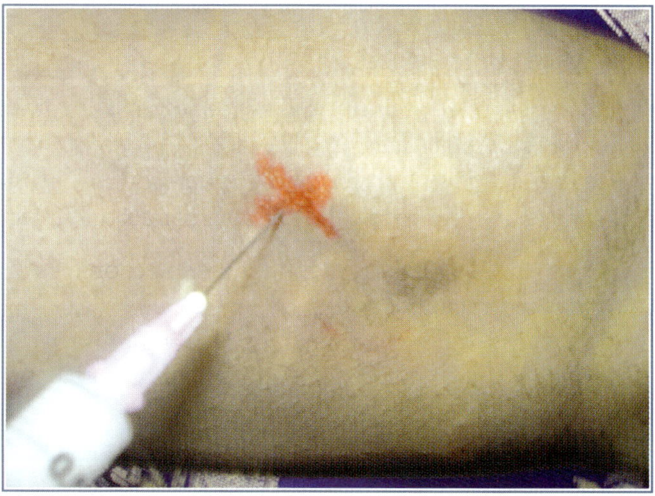

Fig. 4.15B: Insert the needle horizontally towards this point

- Ecchymosis
- Haematoma formation.

Note: The incidence of ecchymosis and haematoma formation can be reduced if immediately after the injection, a firm sterile pressure bandage is applied.

Vital facts: Strictly observe the following after the injection:
- Simple analgesics and NSAIDs are advised
- To prevent the exacerbation of pain, avoid heat and gentle range of motion exercises for few days
- Avoid vigorous exercises for few days to prevent increase in pain.

BURSAE AROUND THE KNEE

Suprapatellar Bursitis

Suprapatellar bursa as the name suggests lies above the patella within the quadriceps femoris muscles. This bursa could have a single or multiple sacs.

Causes

- Acute direct trauma to the front of the knee
- Overuse injuries
- Repeated micro trauma
- Job requiring crawling on the knees (e.g. Housemaid's, carpet layers, etc)
- Calcification of the bursa due to chronic injuries.

Presentation

- Pain in the anterior knee above the patella
- Pain could radiate superiorly into the distal anterior thigh

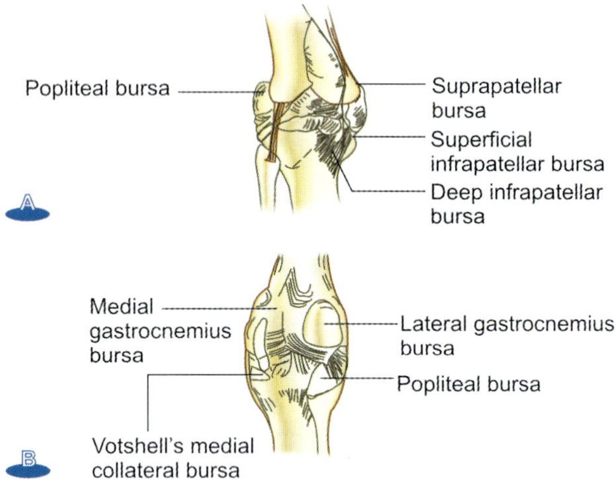

Fig. 4.16: Bursae around the knee

- Patient is unable to kneel or walk down stairs
- With active range of movements especially during first rising, patient could complain of a sharp catching sensation.

Clinical Findings

- Point tenderness just above the patella in the anterior knee
- Passive flexion and active resisted extension of the knee reproduces the pain
- While doing the above manoevre, sudden release of resistance significantly increases the pain
- There could be a swelling in the suprapatellar region with a boggy feel.

Investigations

- Laboratory tests
- Plain X-ray—to rule out occult bony pathology and tumor
- MRI scan
- EMG helps differentiate between femoral neuropathy and lumbar radiculopathy
- Radionucleotide bone scanning to rule out stress fractures
- Injection techniques are both diagnostic and therapeutic.

Procedures

- Position: Supine with a small pillow beneath the knee to slightly flex the knee
- Drugs: 2 ml of 0.25 per cent preservative free bupivacaine and 40 mg of methylprednisolone
- Syringe: 5 ml/1 ½ inches/ 25-gauge needle.

Techniques

- In the position mentioned above, the part is painted and draped
- Push the patella to the medial side
- Identify the superior margin of the patella on the medial side
- Carefully insert the needle horizontally beneath the quadriceps tendon just above the point mentioned previously

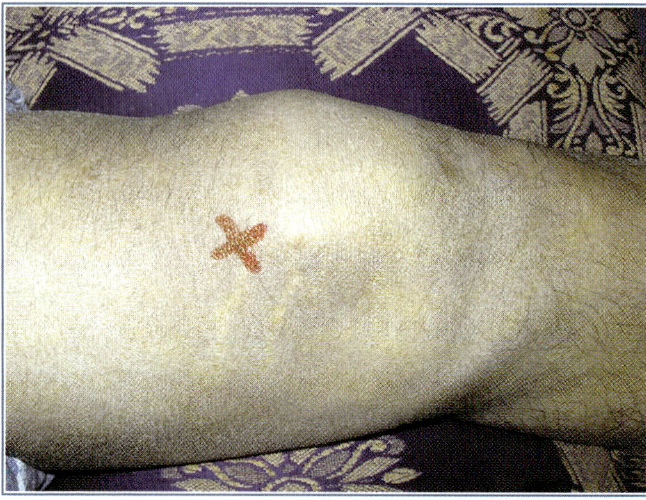

Fig. 4.17A: Mark the superomedial margin of the patella

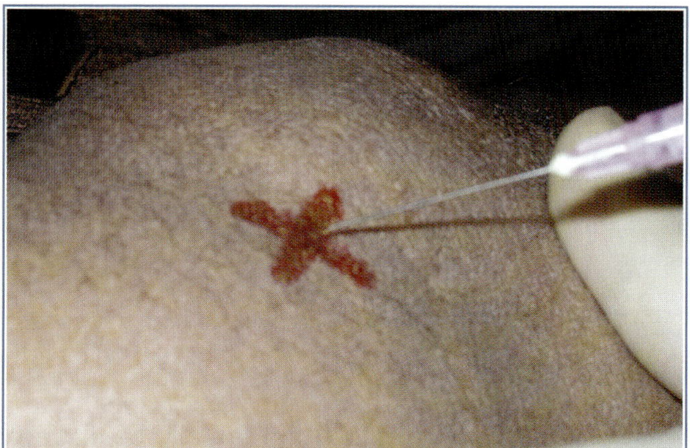

Fig. 4.17B: Insert the needle horizontally beneath the quadriceps tendon at the marked point

- If you hit the bone, withdraw the needle and redirect it more anteriorly
- Advance the needle carefully into the joint space
- Inject the contents of the syringe gently.

Resistance vs Inference

- If there is limited resistance; congratulations, you have hit the right spot
- If there is significant resistance; sorry, you are in the wrong space. Withdraw the needle, redirect and inject.

After care: At the injection site, after the injection

- Apply icepacks
- Apply a firm sterile bandage under pressure.

Complications

- Infection (hence follow strict aseptic measures)
- Transient increase of pain (seen in 25% of the cases)
- Ecchymosis
- Haematoma formation.

Note: The incidence of ecchymosis and haematoma formation can be reduced if immediately after the injection, a firm sterile pressure bandage is applied.

Vital facts: Strictly observe the following after the injection:

- Simple analgesics and NSAIDs are advised
- To prevent the exacerbation of pain, avoid heat and gentle range of motion exercises for few days
- Avoid vigorous exercises for few days to prevent increase in pain.

Prepatellar Bursitis

Prepatellar bursa as the name suggests lies between the subcutaneous tissues and the patella. This bursa could have a single or multiple sacs.

Causes

- Acute direct trauma to the front of the knee
- Overuse injuries
- Repeated micro trauma
- Job requiring crawling on the knees (e.g. Housemaid's, carpet layers, etc)
- Calcification of the bursa due to chronic injuries.

Presentation

- Pain and swelling over the anterior knee and the patella
- Pain could radiate superiorly and inferiorly over the knee
- Patient is unable to kneel or walk down stairs
- With active range of movements especially during first rising, patient could complain of a sharp catching sensation.

Clinical Findings

- Point tenderness over the anterior knee just above the patella
- Swelling over the front of the knee
- Passive flexion and active resisted extension of the knee reproduces the pain

- While doing the above manoeuvre, sudden release of resistance significantly increases the pain
- There could be a swelling in the prepatellar region with a boggy feel.

Investigations

- Laboratory tests
- Plain X-ray—to rule out occult bony pathology and tumour
- MRI scan
- EMG helps to differentiate between femoral neuropathy and lumbar radiculopathy
- Radionucleotide bone scanning to rule out stress fractures
- Injection techniques are both diagnostic and therapeutic.

Procedures

- Position: Supine with a small pillow beneath the knee to slightly flex the knee
- Drugs: 2 ml of 0.25 per cent preservative free bupivacaine and 40 mg of methylprednisolone
- Syringe: 5 ml/1 ½ inches/ 25-gauge needle.

Techniques

- In the position mentioned above, the part is painted and draped
- Identify the center of the patella on the medial side

- Carefully Insert the needle horizontally and subcutaneous into the pre-patellar bursa which is anterior and inferior to patella.
- If you hit the bone, withdraw the needle and redirect it more anteriorly
- Inject the contents of the syringe gently.

Resistance vs Inference

- If there is limited resistance; congratulations, you have hit the right spot
- If there is significant resistance; sorry, you are in the wrong space. Withdraw the needle, redirect and inject.

After care: At the injection site, after the injection

- Apply icepacks
- Apply a firm sterile bandage under pressure.

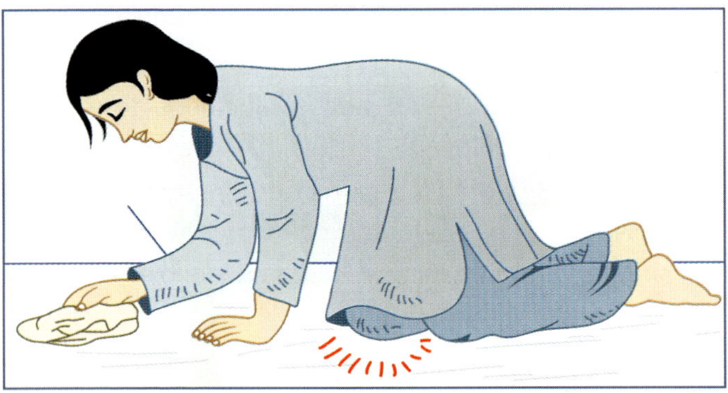

Fig. 4.18A: Showing the mechanism of origin of a prepatellar bursitis in a house maid who kneels heavily against the ground while mopping the floor

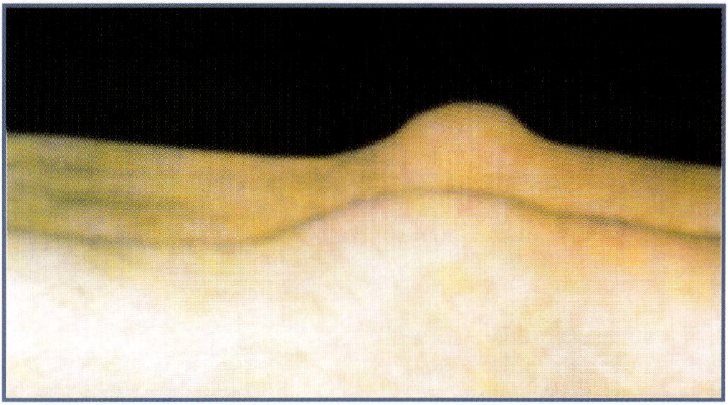

Fig. 4.18B: Clinical photograph of a prepatellar bursitis

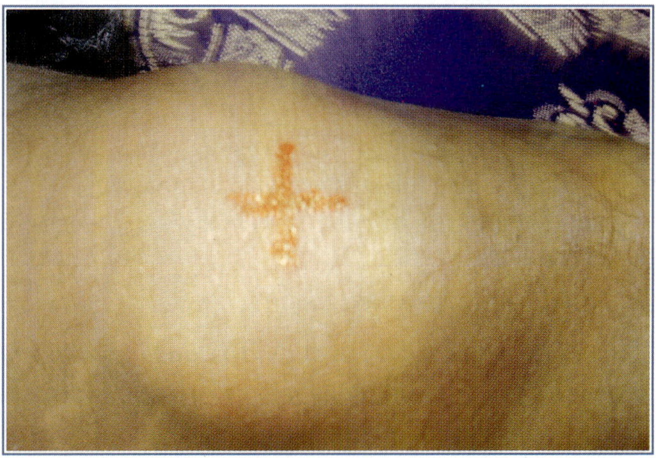

Fig. 4.18C: Identify the center of the patella and mark it with a sterile marker

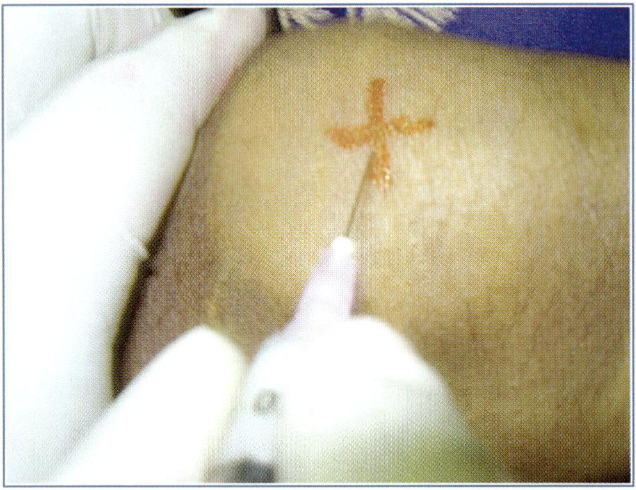

Fig. 4.18D: Insert the needle horizontally through this point into the bursa

Complications

- Infection (hence follow strict aseptic measures)
- Transient increase of pain (seen in 25% of the cases)
- Ecchymosis
- Haematoma formation.

Note: The incidence of ecchymosis and haematoma formation can be reduced if immediately after the injection, a firm sterile pressure bandage is applied.

Vital facts: Strictly observe the following after the injection:
- Simple analgesics and NSAIDs are advised
- To prevent the exacerbation of pain, avoid heat and gentle range of motion exercises for few days
- Avoid vigorous exercises for few days to prevent increase in pain.

Infrapatellar Bursitis

There is two-infrapatellar bursitis, namely superficial and deep. The superficial one lies inbetween the subcutaneous tissue and upper part of ligament patella while the deep one lies between the ligament patellae and tibia.

Causes

- Acute direct trauma to the front of the knee, patella fractures, etc
- Due to overuse injuries (e.g. long distance running, etc)
- Repeated micro-trauma
- Job requiring crawling on the knees (e.g. Housemaid's, carpet layers, etc)
- Calcification of the bursa due to chronic injuries.

Presentation

- Pain and swelling over the front part of the knee below the patella
- Pain could radiate below the knee
- Patient is unable to kneel or walk down stairs
- With active range of movements especially during first rising, patient could complain of a sharp catching sensation.

Clinical Findings

- Point tenderness below the anterior knee just below the patella
- Swelling over the front of the knee near the lower patella

- Passive flexion and active resisted extension of the knee reproduces the pain
- While doing the above manoevre, sudden release of resistance significantly increases the pain
- There could be a swelling in the infrapatellar region with a boggy feel.

Investigations

- Laboratory tests
- Plain X-ray—to rule out occult bony pathology and tumour
- MRI scan
- EMG helps differentiate between femoral neuropathy and lumbar radiculopathy
- Radionucleotide bone scanning to rule out stress fractures
- Injection techniques are both diagnostic and therapeutic.

Procedures

- Position: Supine with a small pillow beneath the knee to slightly flex the knee
- Drugs: 2 ml of 0.25 per cent preservative free bupivacaine and 40 mg of methylprednisolone
- Syringe: 5 ml/1 ½ inches/ 25-gauge needle.

Techniques

- In the position mentioned above, the part is painted and draped

- Identify the centre of the lower pole of the patella on the medial lower margin of the patella for deep bursa.
- Just below this point, Carefully Insert the needle at a 45 degrees angle to the skin to slide into superficial infrapatellar bursa and for deep infrapatellar bursa insert the needle at 90 degree for the skin
- If the needle hits the patella, withdraw and redirect it in a more inferior trajectory
- Now inject the contents of the syringe gently into the bursa.

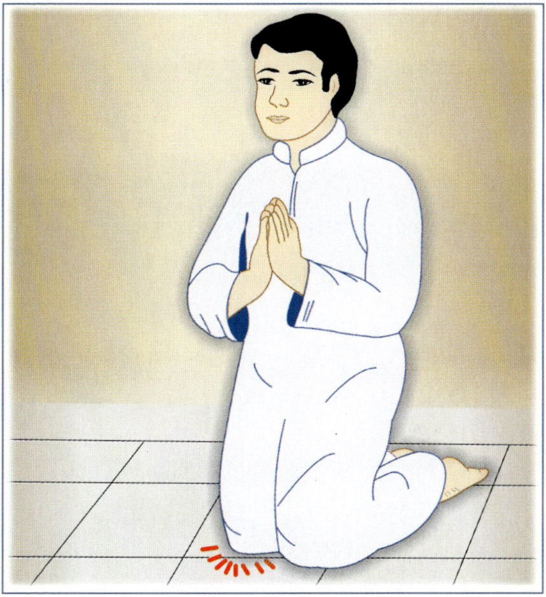

Fig. 4.19A: Showing the mechanism of origin of a infrapatellar bursitis in a clergy who kneels heavily against the ground while praying

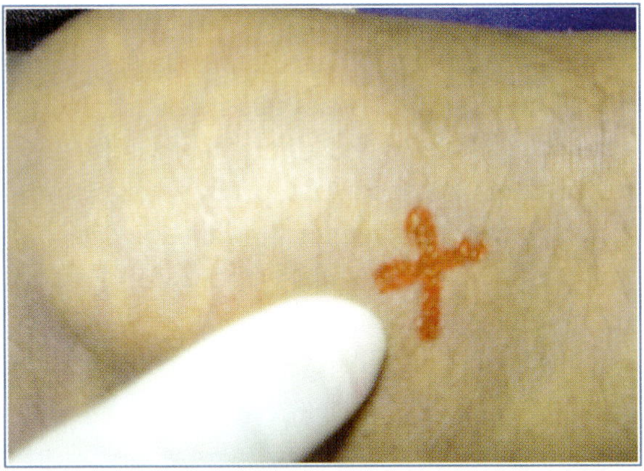

Fig. 4.19B: Identify the center of the lower pole of the patella on the medial side and mark it with a sterile marker

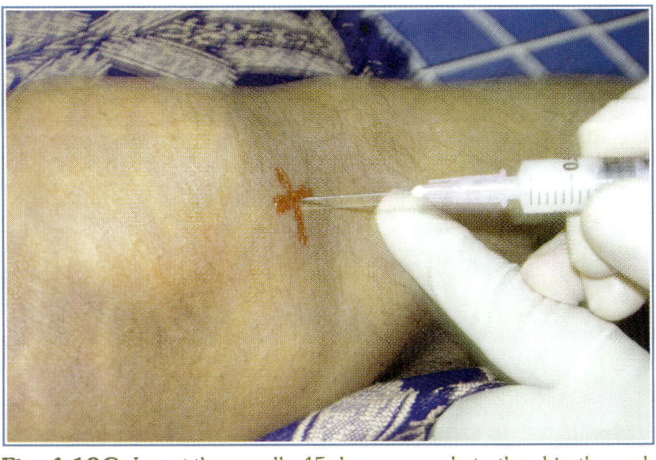

Fig. 4.19C: Insert the needle 45 degrees angle to the skin through this point for the superficial bursa and 90 degrees for the deep bursa

Resistance vs Inference

- If there is limited resistance; congratulations, you have hit the right spot
- If there is significant resistance; sorry, you are in the wrong space. Withdraw the needle, redirect and inject.

After care: At the injection site, after the injection

- Apply icepacks
- Apply a firm sterile bandage under pressure.

Complications

- Infection (hence follow strict aseptic measures)
- Transient increase of pain (seen in 25% of the cases)
- Ecchymosis
- Haematoma formation.

Note: The incidence of ecchymosis and haematoma formation can be reduced if immediately after the injection, a firm sterile pressure bandage is applied.

Vital facts: Strictly observe the following after the injection:

- Simple analgesics and NSAIDs are advised
- To prevent the exacerbation of pain, avoid heat and gentle range of motion exercises for few days
- Avoid vigorous exercises for few days to prevent increase in pain.

Popliteal Bursitis

This was first described by Adam in the year 1840 and later by Baker in 1877. It is a distended bursa in the popliteal fossa and its exact origin is unknown. It is due to the herniation of the synovial membrane through a rent in the capsule.

Causes

- Acute direct trauma to the back of the knee
- Rheumatoid arthritis
- Intra-articular pathology within the knee joint like osteoarthritis, etc.

Presentation

- Pain and swelling over the back of the knee
- Pain could radiate below the knee
- There could be a feeling of stiffness and giving way
- There could be pain in the calf muscle if the bursa ruptures.

Clinical Findings

- There could be a swelling in the popliteal fossa with a boggy feel
- It becomes prominent on extension of the knee and disappears on flexion
- Fluctuation test is positive
- Trans-illumination test is positive.

Investigations

- Laboratory tests
- Plain X-ray to rule out occult bony pathology and tumour

- MRI scan
- Arthrography.

Procedures

- Position: Prone
- Drugs: 2 ml of 0.25 per cent preservative free bupivacaine and 40 mg of methylprednisolone
- Syringe: 5 ml/1½ inches/25-gauge needle.

Techniques

- In the position mentioned above, the part is painted and draped
- Identify the center of the bursa in the popliteal fossa and mark it with a sterile marker
- Carefully insert the needle at the marked point
- If the needle hits the bone, withdraw and redirect it
- Now inject the contents of the syringe gently into the bursa.

Resistance vs Inference

- If there is limited resistance; congratulations, you have hit the right spot.
- If there is significant resistance; sorry, you are in the wrong space. Withdraw the needle, redirect and inject.

After Care

At the injection site, after the injection

- Apply icepacks
- Apply a firm sterile bandage under pressure.

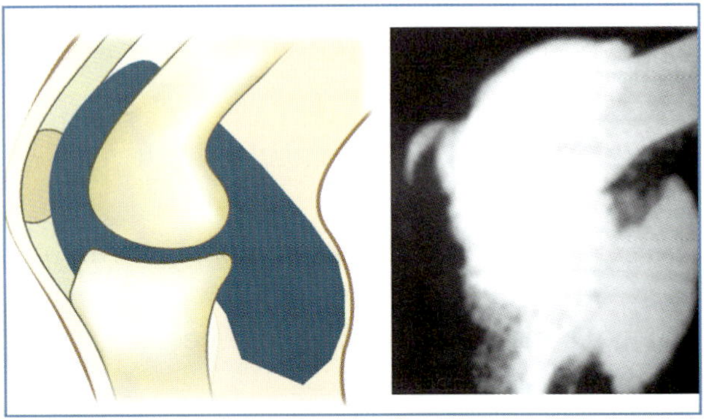

Fig. 4.20A: Showing the popliteal cyst and arthrographic picture of the cyst

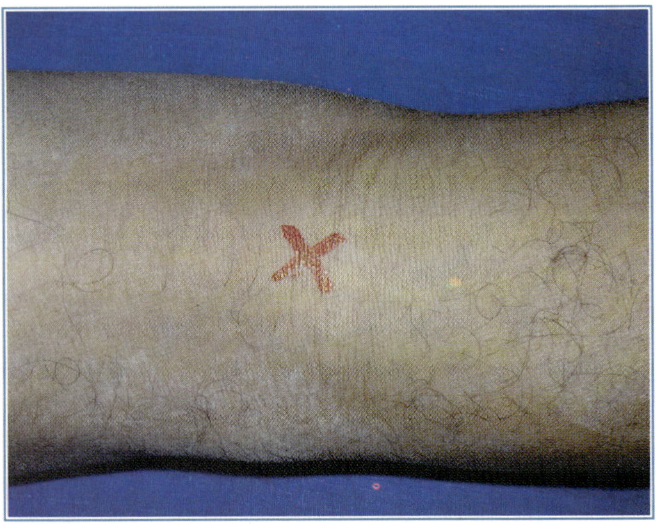

Fig. 4.20B: Mark the most tender point of the cyst in the popliteal cyst

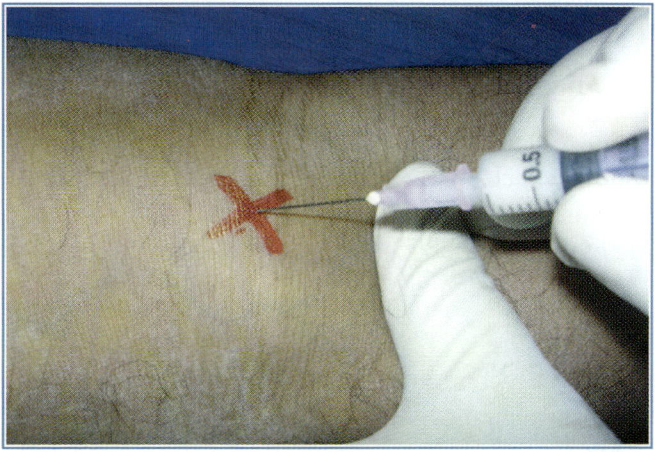

Fig. 4.20C: Insert the needle perpendicular to the skin into the cyst

Complications

- Infection (hence follow strict aseptic measures).
- Transient increase of pain (seen in 25% of the cases).
- Ecchymosis
- Haematoma formation.
- Injury to the popliteal vessels and nerves.

Notes: The incidence of ecchymosis and haematoma formation can be reduced if immediately after the injection, a firm sterile pressure bandage is applied.

Vital facts: Strictly observe the following after the injection:

- Simple analgesics and NSAIDs are advised.
- To prevent the exacerbation of pain, avoid heat and gentle range of motion exercises for few days
- Avoid vigrous exercises for few days to prevent increase in pain.

MISCELLANEOUS

Pes Anserine Bursitis Pain

The pes anserine bursa lies beneath the pes anserine tendon, which is the combined tendon of insertion of sartorius, gracilix and semitendinosus muscle on the medial side of the upper tibia.

Causes

- Acute direct trauma to the medial side of the knee
- Overuse injuries
- Misuse injuries.

Presentation

- Pain and swelling over the medial knee joint
- Pain increases on valgus and external rotation
- Patient is unable to kneel or walk down stairs
- Pain is constant and dull aching in nature
- Pain interferes with sleep
- Chronicity results in calcification of the bursa.

Clinical Findings

- Point tenderness below the medial joint line near the insertion of pes anserine
- Swelling
- Active resisted flexion of the knee reproduces the pain
- While doing the above manoevre, sudden release of resistance significantly increases the pain.

Investigations

- Laboratory tests
- Plain X-ray—to rule out occult bony pathology and tumour
- MRI scan
- EMG helps differentiate between femoral neuropathy and lumbar radiculopathy
- Radio nucleotide bone scanning to rule out stress fractures
- Injection techniques are both diagnostic and therapeutic.

Procedures

- Position: Supine with a small pillow beneath the knee to slightly flex the knee
- Drugs: 2 ml of 0.25 per cent preservative free bupivacaine and 40 mg of methylprednisolone
- Syringe: 5 ml/1 ½ inches/ 25-gauge needle.

Techniques

- In the position mentioned above, the part is painted and draped
- Identify the pes anserine tendon by instructing the patient to flex the knee against resistance
- The point distal to the medial joint space at which the pes anserine tendon attaches to the tibia is the tendon of pes anserine bursa. The bursa is usually identified by point tenderness at that spot

- Carefully insert the needle at an angle of 45 degrees to the tibia
- If you hit the bone, withdraw the needle slightly and redirect it
- Inject the contents of the syringe gently.

Resistance vs Inference

- If there is limited resistance; congratulations, you have hit the right spot
- If there is significant resistance; sorry, you are in the wrong space. Withdraw the needle, redirect and inject.

After care: At the injection site, after the injection:
- Apply icepacks
- Apply a firm sterile bandage under pressure.

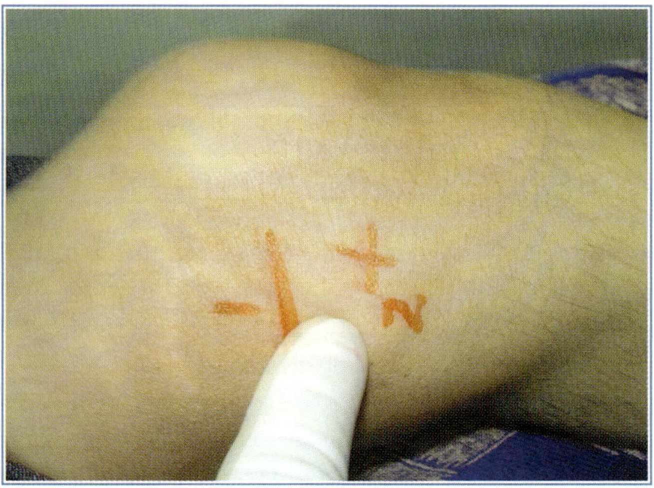

Fig. 4.21A: Mark the medial joint line (Mark 1). Mark 2 indicates the insertion of the pes anserine tendon

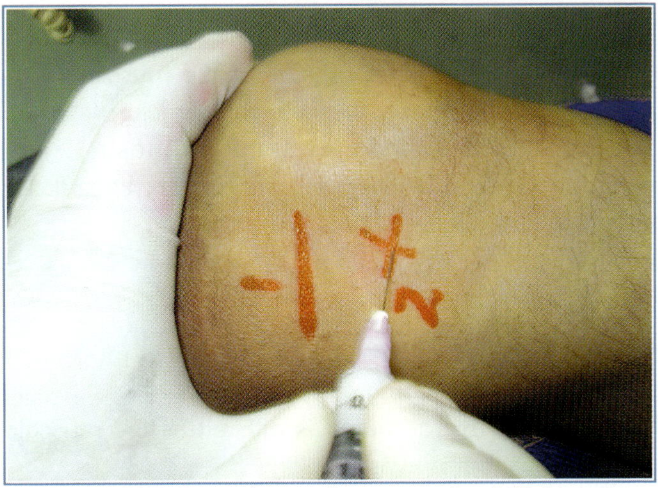

Fig. 4.21B: Insert the needle at an angle of 45 degrees to the skin

Complications

- Infection (hence follow strict aseptic measures)
- Transient increase of pain (seen in 25% of the cases)
- Ecchymosis
- Haematoma formation.

Note: The incidence of ecchymosis and haematoma formation can be reduced if immediately after the injection, a firm sterile pressure bandage is applied.

Vital facts: Strictly observe the following after the injection:
- Simple analgesics and NSAIDs are advised
- To prevent the exacerbation of pain, avoid heat and gentle range of motion exercises for few days
- Avoid vigorous exercises for few days to prevent increase in pain.

Hamstring Tendinitis

The hamstrings muscles consists of the muscles of the posterior compartment of the thigh; namely the biceps femoris, adductor magnus semitendinosus, semimembranosus and BASS. They are primary knee flexors and are inserted into the tibia or fibula.

Reasons for Tendinitis

- Knee is subjected to significant repetitive movements during weight bearing
- Healing of micro-trauma is difficult as the musculotendinous unit is avascular.

Causes

- Acute direct trauma
- Overuse injuries
- Misuse.

Predisposing Factors

- Long distance running
- Dancing activities
- Use of exercise equipments.

Presentation

- Pain over the tendinous insertion
- Pain is constant, severe and interferes with sleep
- Patient holds the knee in a slightly flexed position

- Tenderness is present over the medial portion of the insertion
- Crepitus can be felt on moving the tendon
- Decreased range of movements
- With active range of movements especially during first rising, patient could complain of a sharp catching sensation
- Long standing cases muscle wasting may be seen.

Investigations

- Laboratory tests
- Plain X-ray—to rule out occult bony pathology and tumor
- MRI scan
- EMG helps differentiate between femoral neuropathy and lumbar radiculopathy
- Radionucleotide bone scanning to rule out stress fractures
- Injection techniques are both diagnostic and therapeutic.

Procedures

- Position: Prone with the knee in a slightly flexed position with the anterior ankle resting on a folded towel
- Drugs: 2 ml of 0,25 per cent preservative free bupivacaine and 40 mg of methylprednisolone
- Syringe: 5 ml/ 2 inches/ 25-gauge needle.

Techniques

- In the position mentioned above, the part is painted and draped
- Identify the origin of the hamstrings tendon by asking the patient to flex the knee against the resistance. Mark this point.
- Carefully insert the needle at right angles to the skin towards the origin of the affected tendon.
- Advance the needle till you hit the bone
- Withdraw the needle slightly
- Do an aspiration test and check for paraesthesia in the distribution of the common peroneal and tibial nerve
- If both the test are negative, inject the contents of the syringe gently.

Resistance vs Inference

- If there is limited resistance; congratulations, you have hit the right spot
- If there is significant resistance; sorry, you are in the wrong space. Withdraw the needle, redirect and inject.

After care: At the injection site, after the injection

- Apply icepacks
- Apply a firm sterile bandage under pressure.

Complications

- Infection (hence follow strict aseptic measures)
- Transient increase of pain (seen in 25% of the cases)
- Ecchymosis
- Haematoma formation.

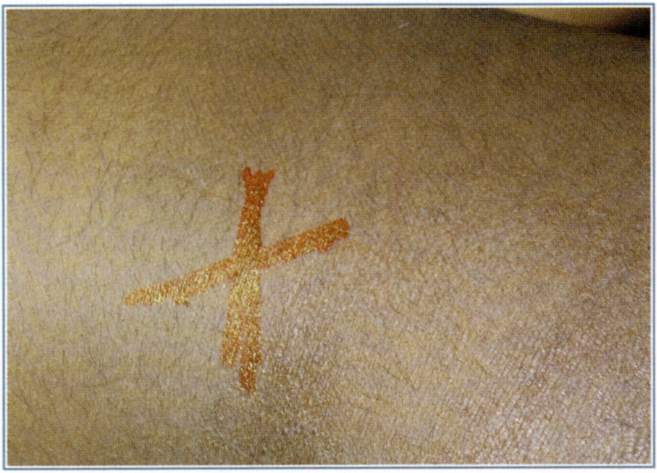

Fig. 4.22A: Identify the origin of the tendon of the hamstrings and mark it with a sterile marker

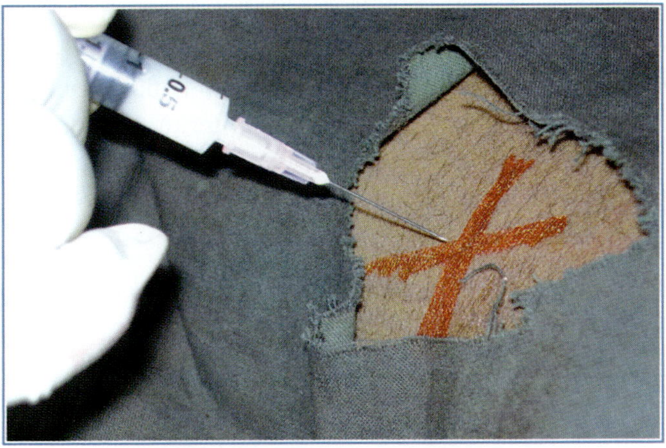

Fig. 4.22B: Insert the needle perpendicular to the skin through this point

Note: The incidence of ecchymosis and haematoma formation can be reduced if immediately after the injection, a firm sterile pressure bandage is applied.

Vital facts: Strictly observe the following after the injection:

- Simple analgesics and NSAIDs are advised
- To prevent the exacerbation of pain, avoid heat and gentle range of motion exercises for few days
- Avoid vigorous exercises for few days to prevent increase in pain.

ANKLE JOINT AND FOOT COMPLEX

Though there are several approaches to the ankle, the one that is most commonly employed is the anterior approach and it consists of the following steps:

- The foot is in moderate plantar flexion
- Insert the needle between the talus and tibia bounded medially between the tibialis anterior tendon and laterally by the extensor hallucis longus tendon
- Direct the needle tangentially towards the curve of the talus.

Note: The most common mistake is to direct the needle too much towards the heel.

INTRA-ARTICULAR INJECTIONS

Ankle Joint

Arthritis is the most common cause of pain in the ankle joint.

Causes

- Osteoarthrtis
- Rheumatoid arthritis
- Post-traumatic osteoarthritis.

Less Common Causes

- Collagen vascular diseases
- Infection
- Villonodular synovitis.

Presentation

- Pain is localized around the ankle and distal leg
- Movements of the ankle more so the dorsiflexion makes the pain worse
- Rest and heat decreases the pain
- Pain interferes with sleep
- Grating, crepitus, popping sensation, etc. are the other complaints
- Day do day activities like walking, standing, climbing, etc. are affected
- Muscle wasting of the leg and frozen ankle are the effects of prolonged arthritis.

Investigations

- Laboratory tests
- Plain X-ray—to rule out occult bony pathology and tumour
- MRI scan
- Injection techniques are both diagnostic and therapeutic.

Procedures

- Position: Supine position with the foot in the neutral position
- Drugs: 2 ml of 0.25 per cent preservative free bupivacaine and 40 mg of methylprednisolone
- Syringe: 5 ml/ 2 inches/ 25-gauge needle.

Techniques

- In the position mentioned above, the part is painted and draped
- Identify the junction of the tibia and fibula just above the talus
- At the above mentioned point there is a triangular indentation that indicates the joint space.

  Next identity the anterior and posterior landmarks. The anterior one is the medial border of tibialis anterior tendon and the posterior landmark is the anterior border of medial malleolus.
- Mark this point.
- Carefully advance the needle into the joint through this point in a postero-lateral direction.
- If you hit the bone withdraw the needle slightly and redirect it more superiorly and medially
- Inject the contents of the syringe gently into the joint.

Resistance vs Inference

- If there is limited resistance; congratulations, you have hit the right spot

- If there is significant resistance; sorry, you are in the wrong space. Withdraw the needle, redirect and inject.

After care: At the injection site, after the injection
- Apply icepacks
- Apply a firm sterile bandage under pressure.

Complications

- Infection (hence follow strict aseptic measures)
- Transient increase of pain (seen in 25% of the cases)
- Ecchymosis
- Haematoma formation.

Note: The incidence of ecchymosis and haematoma formation can be reduced if immediately after the injection, a firm sterile pressure bandage is applied.

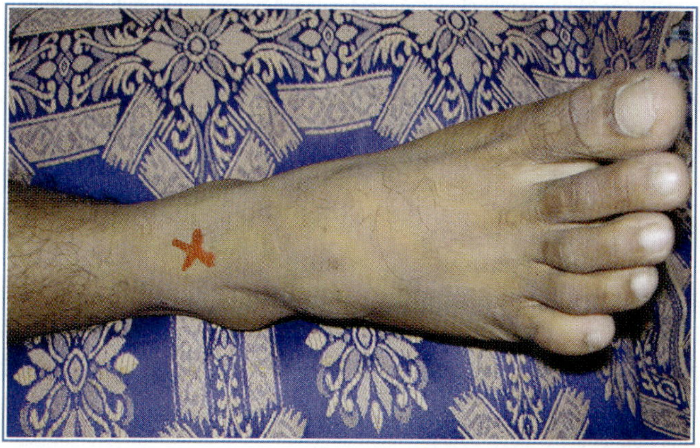

Fig. 4.23A: Identify the junction of the tibia and fibula just above the talus and mark it with a sterile marker. This point corresponds to a triangular indentation that marks the ankle joint

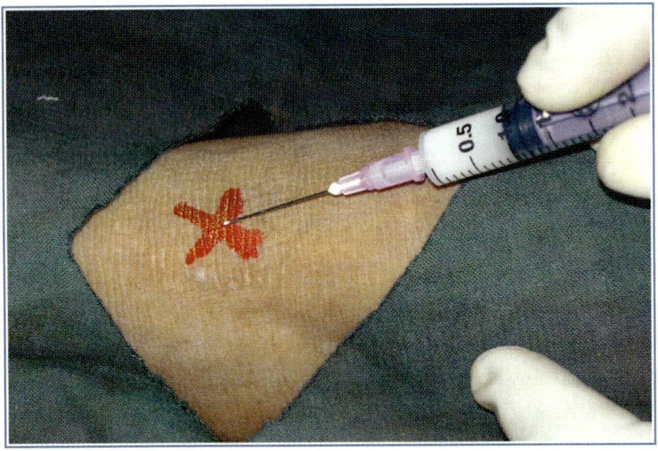

Fig. 4.23B: Insert the needle into the joint through this point in a postero-lateral direction

Vital facts: Strictly observe the following after the injection:
- Simple analgesics and NSAIDs are advised
- To prevent the exacerbation of pain, avoid heat and gentle range of motion exercises for few days
- Avoid vigorous exercises for few days to prevent increase in pain.

The Subtalar Joint

The posterior subtalar joint often communicates with the ankle joint particularly in rheumatoid arthritis. Hence specific injection into this joint is not needed. The approach commonly used is the lateral approach and it consists of the following steps:

- Patient is in prone position
- Draw a horizontal line one inch above the distal end of the lateral malleolus

- Draw another line 1 cm from the posterior border of the shaft of the fibula
- The point where these two lines cross marks the site of entry

Arthritis is the most common cause of pain in the subtalar joint.

Causes

- Osteoarthrtis
- Rheumatoid arthritis
- Post-traumatic osteoarthritis.

Less Common Causes

- Collagen vascular diseases
- Infection
- Villonodular synovitis.

Presentation

- Pain is felt deep in the heel
- Movements especially adduction of the calcaneus makes the pain worse
- Rest and heat decreases the pain
- Pain is constant and dull aching and interferes with sleep
- Grating, crepitus, popping sensation, etc. are the other complaints
- Day do day activities like walking, standing, climbing, etc. are painful and difficult
- Muscle wasting of the leg and frozen ankle are the effects of prolonged arthritis.

Investigations

- Laboratory tests
- Plain X-ray—to rule out occult bony pathology and tumor
- MRI scan
- Injection techniques are both diagnostic and therapeutic.

Procedures

- Position: Supine position with the leg slightly in abducted position
- Drugs: 2 ml of 0.25 per cent preservative free bupivacaine and 40 mg of methylprednisolone
- Syringe: 5 ml/ 2 inches/ 25-gauge needle.

Techniques

- In the position mentioned above, the part is painted and draped
- Identify the medial malleolus
- Next identify the sustentaculum tali which lies one inch below the medial malleolus
- Locate the subtalar joint which is above and slightly posterior to the sustentaculum tali
- Mark this point.
- Carefully advance the needle into the joint at right angles to the skin
- If you hit the bone withdraw the needle slightly and redirect it more superiorly and anteriorly
- Inject the contents of the syringe gently into the joint.

Resistance vs Inference

- If there is limited resistance; congratulations, you have hit the right spot
- If there is significant resistance; sorry, you are in the wrong space. Withdraw the needle, redirect and inject.

After care: At the injection site, after the injection:

- Apply icepacks
- Apply a firm sterile bandage under pressure.

Complications

- Infection (hence follow strict aseptic measures)
- Transient increase of pain (seen in 25% of the cases)

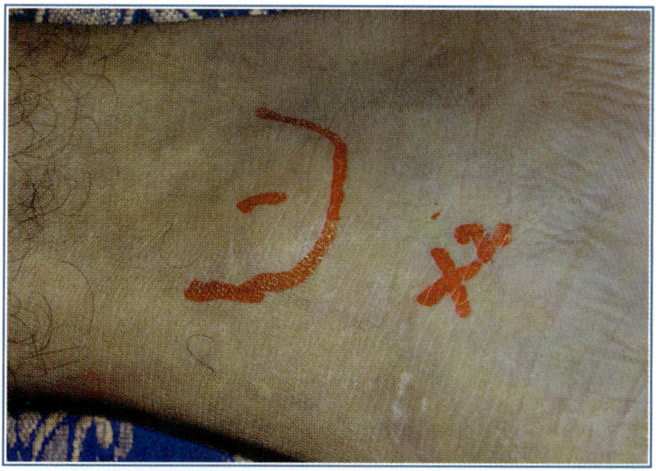

Fig. 4.24A: Identify the medial mallelous and mark it as 1. Now identify the sustentaculum talus which lies one inch below the medial malleolus and mark it as 2

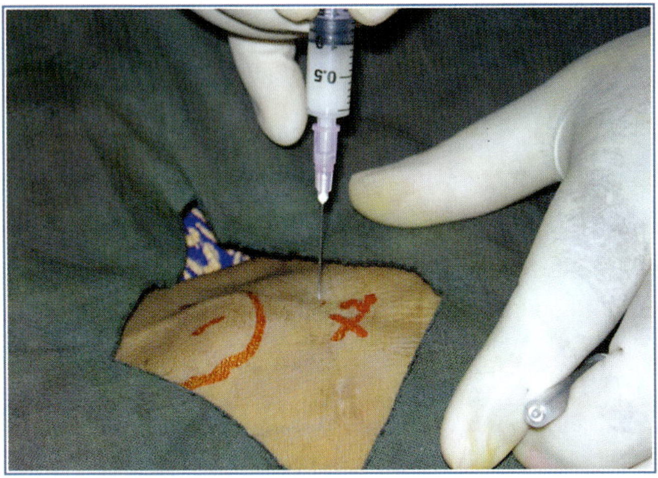

Fig. 4.24B: Insert the needle slightly posterior to the above point

- Ecchymosis
- Haematoma formation.

Note: The incidence of ecchymosis and haematoma formation can be reduced if immediately after the injection, a firm sterile pressure bandage is applied.

Vital facts: Strictly observe the following after the injection:
- Simple analgesics and NSAIDs are advised
- To prevent the exacerbation of pain, avoid heat and gentle range of motion exercises for few days
- Avoid vigorous exercises for few days to prevent increase in pain.

The Midtarsal Joint

Injecting into this joint is difficult. The injection is given into the intertarsal joint space on the dorsum of the foot.

Arthritis is the most common cause of pain in the midtarsal joint.

Causes

- Osteoarthrtis
- Rheumatoid arthritis
- Post-traumatic osteoarthritis.

Less Common Causes

- Collagen vascular diseases
- Infection
- Villonodular synovitis.

Presentation

- Pain is localized to the dorsum of the foot
- Movements of the foot more so the inversion and adduction of the midtarsal joints makes the pain worse
- Rest and heat decreases the pain
- Pain interferes with sleep
- Grating, crepitus, popping sensation, etc are the other complaints
- Simple day-to-day activities like walking, standing, climbing, etc. are affected.

Investigations

- Laboratory tests
- Plain X-ray—to rule out occult bony pathology and tumor
- MRI scan
- Injection techniques are both diagnostic and therapeutic.

Procedures

- *Position:* Supine position with the foot in the neutral position
- Drugs: 2 ml of 0.25 per cent preservative free bupivacaine and 40 mg of methylprednisolone
- *Syringe:* 5 ml/ 2 inches/ 25-gauge needle.

Techniques

- In the position mentioned above, the part is painted and draped
- Identify the midtarsal joint space at the midpoint between navicular and cuneiform bones
- Mark this point.
- Pass the needle at right angles to this joint through this point
- If you hit the bone withdraw the needle slightly and redirect it more superiorly and medially
- Inject the contents of the syringe gently into the joint.

Resistance vs Inference

- If there is limited resistance; congratulations, you have hit the right spot
- If there is significant resistance; sorry, you are in the wrong space. Withdraw the needle, redirect and inject.

After care: At the injection site, after the injection:
- Apply icepacks
- Apply a firm sterile bandage under pressure.

Complications

- Infection (hence follow strict aseptic measures)
- Transient increase of pain (seen in 25% of the cases)
- Ecchymosis
- Haematoma formation.

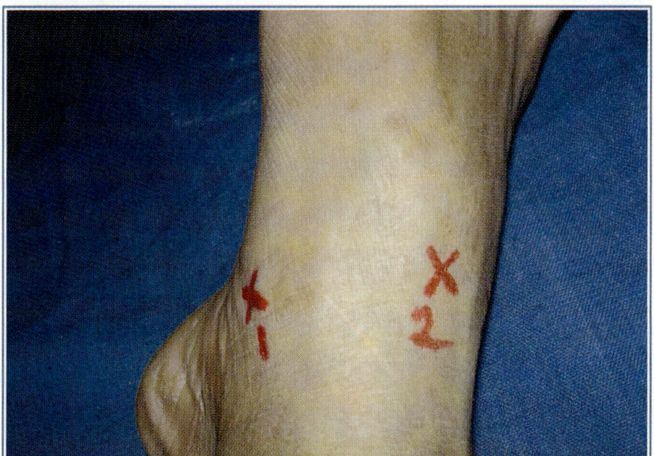

Fig. 4.25A: Identify the navicular bone and mark it as 1. Next identify the cuneiform bone and mark it as 3

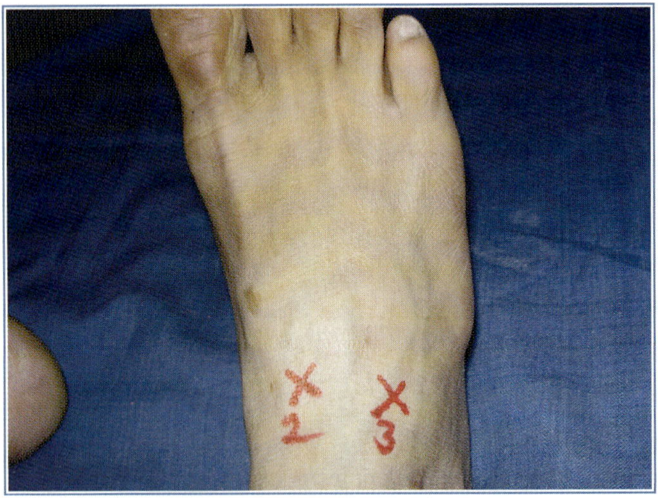

Fig. 4.25B: Now identify the midtarsal joint space that is in between Mark 1 and 3 and mark it as 2

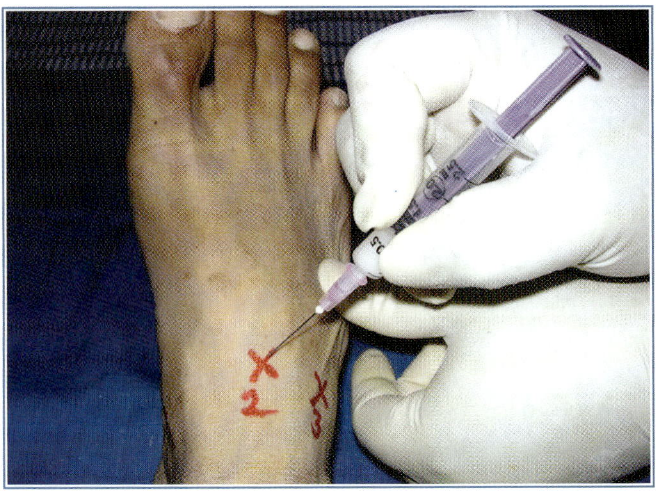

Fig. 4.25C: Pass the needle at right angles to mark 2 into the midtarsal joint

Note: The incidence of ecchymosis and haematoma formation can be reduced if immediately after the injection, a firm sterile pressure bandage is applied.

Vital facts: Strictly observe the following after the injection:
- Simple analgesics and NSAIDs are advised
- To prevent the exacerbation of pain, avoid heat and gentle range of motion exercises for few days
- Avoid vigorous exercises for few days to prevent increase in pain.

The Great Toe

Arthritis is the most common cause of pain within the great toe.

Causes

- Osteoarthrtis
- Rheumatoid arthritis
- Post-traumatic osteoarthritis.

Less Common Causes

- Collagen vascular diseases
- Infection
- Villonodular synovitis.

Presentation

- Pain is localized around the great toe
- Movements of the great toe more so the dorsiflexion increases the pain

- Rest and heat decreases the pain.
- Pain interferes with sleep
- Grating, crepitus, popping sensation, etc are the other complaints
- Day do day activities like walking, standing, climbing etc are affected.

Investigation

- Laboratory tests
- Plain X-ray—to rule out occult bony pathology and tumor
- MRI scan
- Injection techniques are both diagnostic and therapeutic.

Procedures

- Position: Supine position with the foot in the neutral position and knee flexed over a folded towel.
- Drugs: 2 ml of 0.25 per cent preservative free bupivacaine and 40 mg of methylprednisolone
- Syringe: 5 ml/ 2 inches/ 25-gauge needle.

Techniques

- In the position mentioned above, the part is painted and draped
- To open the joint space, distract the affected toe and slightly plantarflex it
- Next identify the joint space, mark it, and insert the needle at right angles to the joint just next to the extensor tendons through the skin

- Mark this point
- Carefully advance the needle into the joint through this point
- Inject the contents of the syringe gently into the joint.

Resistance vs Inference

- If there is limited resistance; congratulations, you have hit the right spot
- If there is significant resistance; sorry, you are in the wrong space. Withdraw the needle, redirect and inject.

After care: At the injection site, after the injection:

- Apply icepacks
- Apply a firm sterile bandage under pressure.

Complications

- Infection (hence follow strict aseptic measures)
- Transient increase of pain (seen in 25% of the cases)
- Ecchymosis
- Haematoma formation.

Note: The incidence of ecchymosis and haematoma formation can be reduced if immediately after the injection, a firm sterile pressure bandage is applied.

Vital facts: Strictly observe the following after the injection:

- Simple analgesics and NSAIDs are advised
- To prevent the exacerbation of pain, avoid heat and gentle range of motion exercises for few days
- Avoid vigorous exercises for few days to prevent increase in pain.

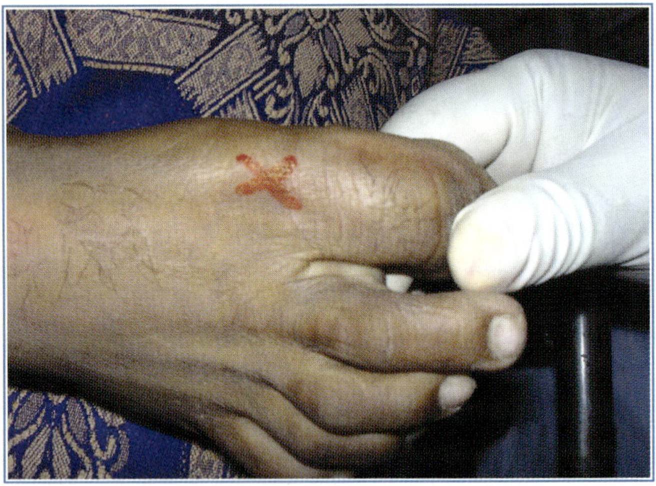

Fig. 4.26A: To open the joint space, distract and plantarflex the great toe. Identify the joint space and mark it with a sterile marker

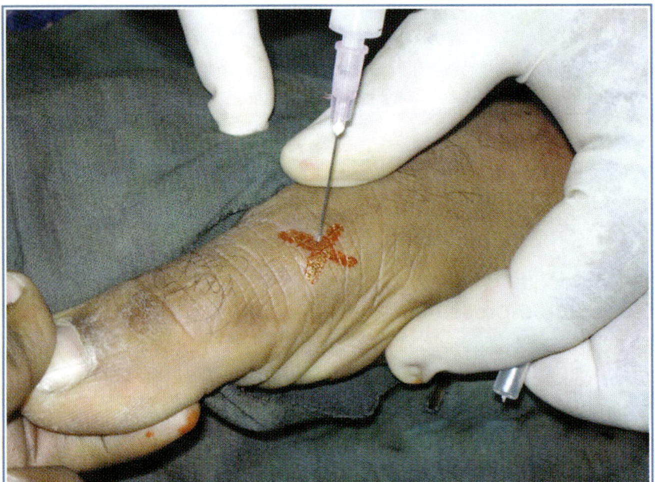

Fig. 4.26B: Insert the needle at right angles to the joint

LOCAL INFILRATION FOR THE SOFT TISSUE LESIONS AROUND THE ANKLE

Deltoid Ligament Sprain

Causes

- Due to sudden over pronation of the ankle
- Due to repetitive microtrauma to the ligament from overuse or misuse, e.g. long distance runners.

Presentation

- Pain is felt must below the medial malleolus
- Ecchymosis over the ligament
- Point tenderness over the medial malleolus
- Plantar flexion and passive eversion increases the pain.

Investigations

- Laboratory tests
- Plain X-ray—to rule out occult bony pathology and tumor
- MRI scan—if there is disruption of the deltoid ligament, joint instability, occult masses, etc
- Injection techniques are both diagnostic and therapeutic.

Procedures

- Position: Supine position with the foot in the neutral position

- Drugs: 2 ml of 0.25 per cent preservative free bupivacaine and 40 mg of methylprednisolone
- Syringe: 5 ml/ 2 inches/ 25-gauge needle.

Techniques

- In the position mentioned above and with the legs slightly adducted, the part is painted and draped
- Identify the lower margin of the medial malleolus
- Mark this point
- Carefully advance the needle through this point at an angle of 30 degrees to the ankle and advance it through the skin till it impinges on the lower margin of the medial malleolus
- Now withdraw the needle slightly and inject the contents of the syringe gently into the joint.

Resistance vs Inferences

- If there is limited resistance; congratulations, you have hit the right spot
- If there is significant resistance; sorry, you are in the wrong space. Withdraw the needle, redirect and inject.

After care: At the injection site, after the injection:
- Apply icepacks
- Apply a firm sterile bandage under pressure.

Complications

- Infection (hence follow strict aseptic measures)
- Transient increase of pain (seen in 25% of the cases)

- Ecchymosis
- Haematoma formation.

Note: The incidence of ecchymosis and haematoma formation can be reduced if immediately after the injection, a firm sterile pressure bandage is applied.

Vital facts: Strictly observe the following after the injection:
- Simple analgesics and NSAIDs are advised
- To prevent the exacerbation of pain, avoid heat and gentle range of motion exercises for few days
- Avoid vigorous exercises for few days to prevent increase in pain.

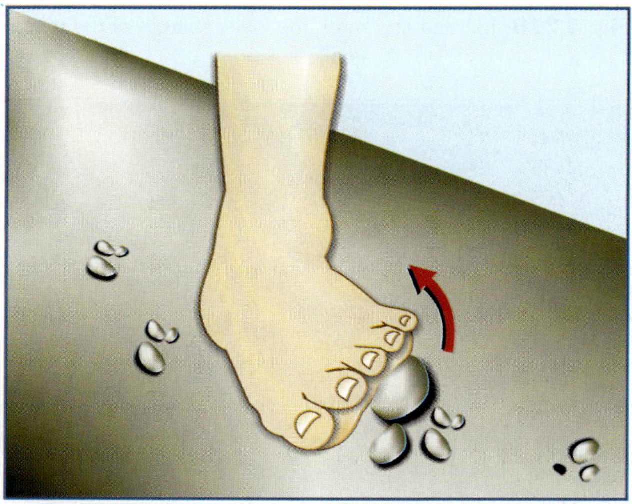

Fig. 4.27A: Eversion injury to the ankle causes deltoid ligament sprain

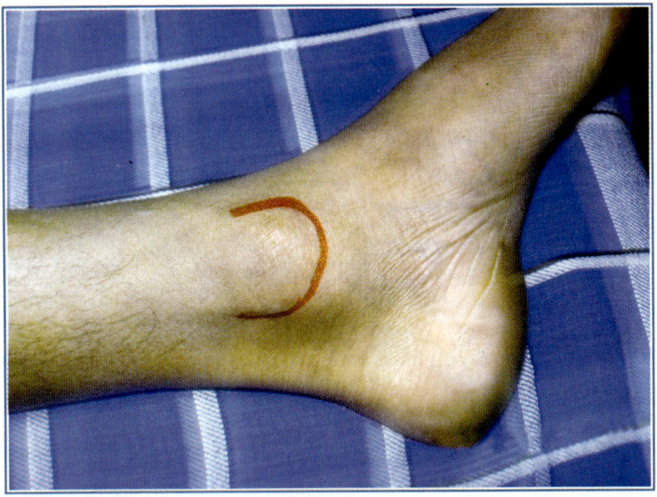

Fig. 4.27B: Identify and mark the lower margin of the medial malleolus

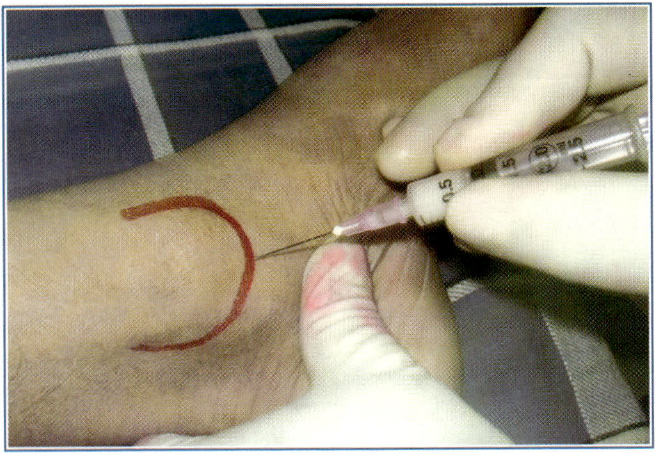

Fig. 4.27C: Insert the needle through this point at an angle of 30 degrees to the ankle

Anterior Talofibular Ligament Strain

Causes

- Sudden forceful inversion injury
- Due to overuse or misuse from long distance running.

Presentation

- Pain below the lateral malleolus
- Inversion of the ankle increases the pain
- Tenderness just below the lateral malleolus
- Ecchymosis over the joint present.

Investigations

- Plain X-ray of the ankle
- Laboratory investigations
- MRI.

Procedures

- Patient is supine
- Keep the lower limb adducted
- Identify the lower margin of the lateral malleolus
- Insert the needle at 30 degrees angle to the ankle to impinge on the lower margin of the lateral malleolus
- Withdraw the needle slightly and inject.

Resistance vs Inference

- Slight resistance; congratulations you have hit the right target

- Significant resistance; sorry, you have missed the target. Slightly withdraw, realign and inject.

After care: At the injection site, after the injection:

- Apply icepacks
- Apply a firm sterile bandage under pressure.

Complications

- Infection (hence follow strict aseptic measures)
- Transient increase of pain (seen in 25% of the cases)
- Ecchymosis
- Haematoma formation.

Note: The incidence of ecchymosis and haematoma formation can be reduced if immediately after the injection, a firm sterile pressure bandage is applied.

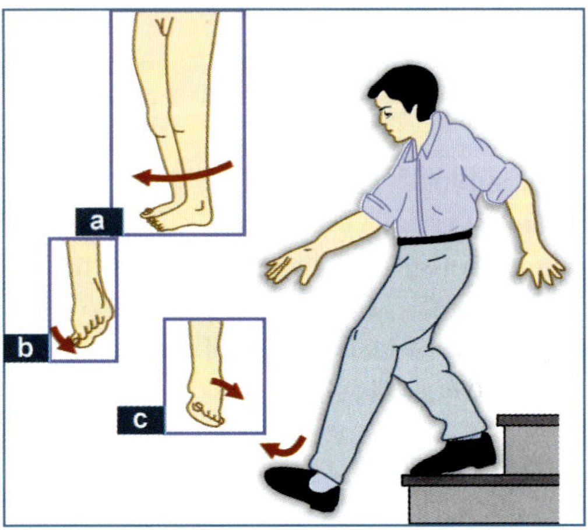

Fig. 4.28A: Inversion injury causes sprain of the anterior talo-fibular ligament of the ankle

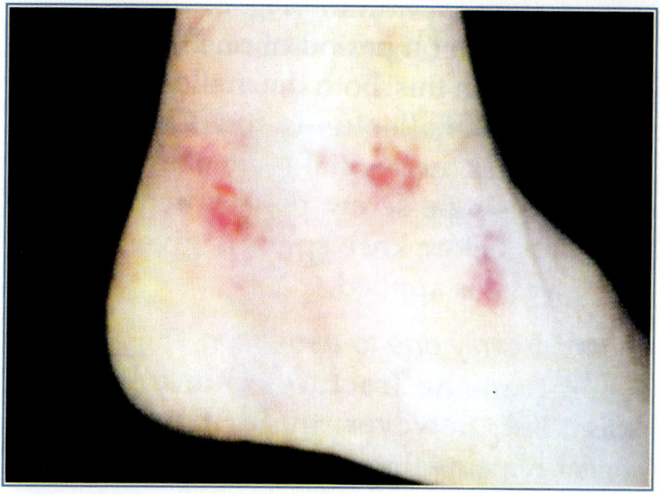

Fig. 4.28B: Clinical photograph of the lateral ankle sprain

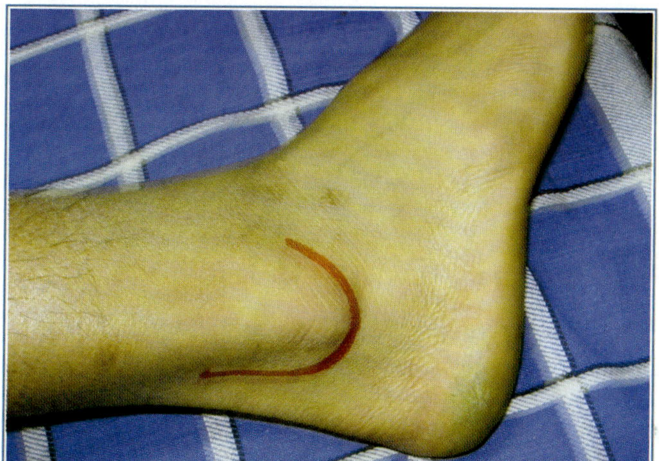

Fig. 4.28C: Identify and mark the lower margin of the lateral malleolus

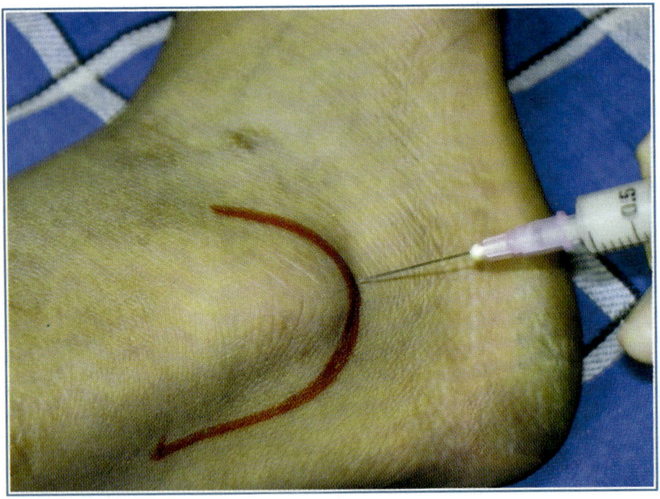

Fig. 4.28D: Insert the needle at 30-degree angle to the lateral malleolus

Vital facts: Strictly observe the following after the injection:
- Simple analgesics and NSAIDs are advised
- To prevent the exacerbation of pain, avoid heat and gentle range of motion exercises for few days
- Avoid vigorous exercises for few days to prevent increase in pain.

Posterior Tarsal Tunnel Syndrome

PTS is due to compression of the posterior tibial nerve as it passes through the posterior tarsal tunnel.

Causes

- Injury to the ankle such as fractures, dislocations, crush injury, etc
- Thrombophlebitis of the posterior tibial artery.

Presentation

- Pain, numbness, paraesthesiae of the sole of the foot
- Pain could radiate proximally towards the medial ankle
- Weakness of the flexors and instability
- Nocturnal foot pain
- Tenderness present over the posterior tibial nerve behind the medial malleolus
- Active inversion of the ankle produces pain.

Differential Diagnosis

- Arthritis of the ankle: X-ray helps to differentiate
- Lumbar radiculopathy: Reflex, motor and sensory changes
- Diabetic neuropathy.

Investigations

- Plain X-ray of the ankle
- Laboratory investigations
- MRI
- EMG
- Injection technique.

Procedures

- Patient is in the lateral decubitus position
- Keep the affected leg in the dependent position with the leg slightly flexed
- Identify the area between the medial malleolus and the Achilles tendon

- Palpate for the posterior tibial artery inbetween these two points
- Insert the needle at this point and direct it anteriorly towards the posterior tibial artery
- If the posterior tibial pulsations cannot be identified, then direct the needle towards the posterior superior border of the medial malleolus
- Advance the needle towards the posterior groove of the medial malleolus towards the posterior tibial nerve.
- If you could elicit a paraesthesiae the distribution of the posterior tibial nerve, you have hit the right spot
- If you fail to elicit the paraesthesiae, withdraw and redirect it slightly more cephalad till a paraesthesia is obtained
- On eliciting the paraesthesiae, withdraw the needle slightly by 1 mm
- With this paraesthesiae should disappear and not persist
- Test aspiration is carried out
- If test aspiration is negative and if there is no persistent paraesthesiae inject 6 ml of the contents of the syringe slowly.

Caution: Do not inject the drugs into the tibial nerve.

Resistance vs Inference

- Slight resistance; congratulation, you have hit the right target.
- Significant resistance; sorry, you have missed the target. Slightly withdraw, realign and inject.

After care: At the injection site, after the injection:

- Apply icepacks
- Apply a firm sterile bandage under pressure.

Complications

- Infection (hence follow strict aseptic measures)
- Transient increase of pain (seen in 25% of the cases)
- Ecchymosis
- Haematoma formation.

Note: The incidence of ecchymosis and haematoma formation can be reduced if immediately after the injection, a firm sterile pressure bandage is applied.

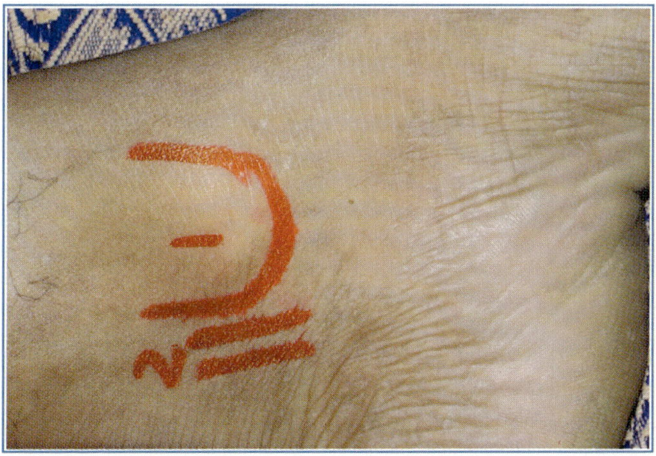

Fig. 4.29A: Identify the medial malleolus (Mark it as 1) and the posterior tibial artery (Mark it as 2) as shown in the figure

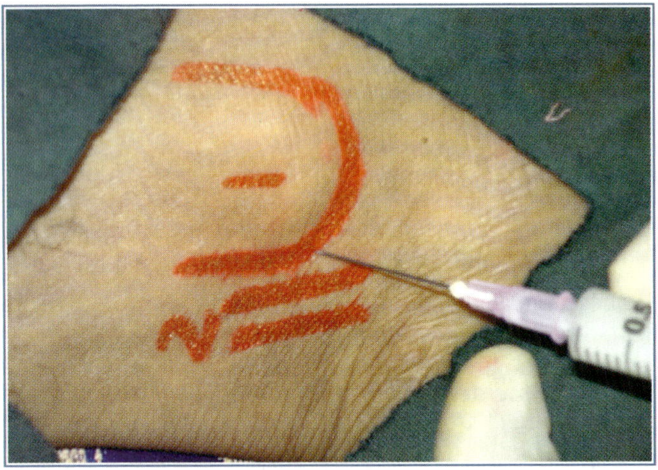

Fig. 4.29B: Advance the needle towards the posterosuperior border of the medial malleolus (Mark 2)

Vital facts: Strictly observe the following after the injection:
- Simple analgesics and NSAIDs are advised
- To prevent the exacerbation of pain, avoid heat and gentle range of motion exercises for few days
- Avoid vigorous exercises for few days to prevent increase in pain.

Achilles Tendinitis

Approach is best from the lateral side of the heel, just above the top of the calcaneum. The needle is directed medially and downwards towards the bursa that lies beneath the skin. Do not inject into the tendon *per se*.

Causes

- Repetitive trauma
- Running, sudden stopping and starting as in tennis
- Repeated overuse and misuse
- Improper stretching of gastrocnemiums and Achilles tendon prior to exercise
- Calcium deposition.

Note: The reasons for susceptibility: Its relative avascularity.

Presentation

- Pain localized to the posterior ankle
- It is continuous and dull aching
- Signifies sleep disturbances
- To avoid plantar flexing the foot, patient assumes a flat-footed gait
- A creaking, grating or crepitus could be heard in the region of tendonachilles on passive plant or flexion
- Later a chronic tendinitis may cause sudden rupture of tendoachilles.

Vital facts: Sites of rupture:
- At insertion on the calcaneus
- 5 cm above its insertion where it is very narrow.

Investigations

- Plain X-ray of the ankle
- Laboratory investigations
- MRI

- EMG
- Injection technique—both diagnostic and therapeutic
- Bone scan—to rule out stress fractures.

Preparation

- Position: Prone
- Drugs: 2 ml of 0.25 per cent preservative free bupivacaine and 40 mg of methylprednisolone
- Syringe: 5 ml/1 ½ inches length and 25-gauge needle.

Procedures

- Patient is in the prone position
- Keep the affected leg in hanging from the edge of a table
- To Identify the margin of the Achilles tendon gently dorsiflex the foot.

Note: This is necessary to avoid injecting directly into the tendon.

- Now identify the most tender point at the tendinous insertion or at its narrowest portion about 5 cm above its insertion. Mark these points with a sterile marker
- Paint and drape the area
- Insert the needle at this point by the side of the tendon.

Caution: Do not enter the substance of the Achilles-tendon.

- Inject the contents of the syringe slowly and gently while the needle is slowly withdrawn.

Resistance vs Inference

- Slight resistance; congratulations you have hit the right target.
- Significant resistance; sorry, you have missed the target. Slightly withdraw, realign and inject.

After care: At the injection site, after the injection:

- Apply icepacks
- Apply a firm sterile bandage under pressure.

Complications

- Infection (hence follow strict aseptic measures)
- Transient increase of pain (seen in 25% of the cases)

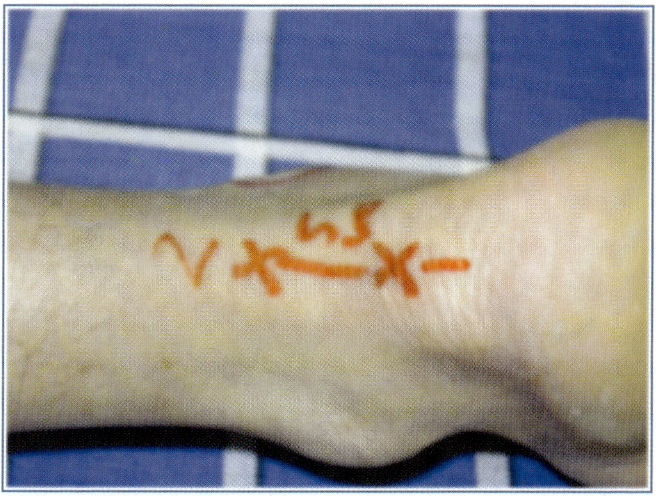

Fig. 4.30A: Identify the insertion of the Achilles tendon and mark it as 1. Mark another point 2 about 5 cm above point 1

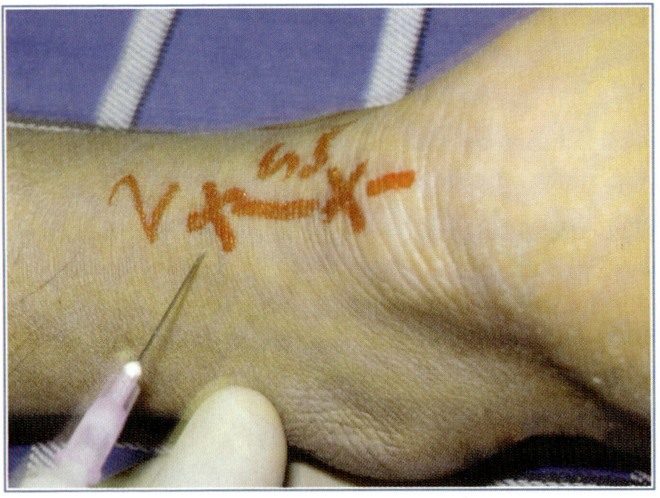

Fig. 4.30B: Insert the needle at point 2 by the side of the tendon

- Ecchymosis
- Haematoma formation.

Note: The incidence of ecchymosis and haematoma formation can be reduced if immediately after the injection, a firm sterile pressure bandage is applied.

Vital facts: Strictly observe the following after the injection:
- Simple analgesics and NSAIDs are advised
- To prevent the exacerbation of pain, avoid heat and gentle range of motion exercises for few days
- Avoid vigorous exercises for few days to prevent increase in pain.

Fibulocalcaneal Ligament Strain

Causes

- Sudden inversion of the ankle
- Repetitive microtrauma.

Presentation

- Pain is felt in the anterior and inferior to the lateral malleolus
- Inversion of the ankle increases the pain
- Point tenderness just below the lateral malleolus
- Ecchymosis is present
- Passive inversion of the ankle increases pain.

Investigations

- Plain X-ray of the ankle
- Laboratory investigations
- MRI
- EMG
- Injection technique—both diagnostic and therapeutic
- Bone scan—to rule out stress fractures.

Preparation

- Position: Prone
- Drugs: 2 ml of 0.25 per cent preservative free bupivacaine and 40 mg of methylprednisolone
- Syringe: 5 ml/1 ½ inches length and 25-gauge needle.

Techniques

- Identify the lower margin of the lateral malleolus
- 1-½ inches below this point, the needle is inserted at a 30-degree angle to the ankle to impinge against the lower margin of the lateral malleolus.
- Withdraw the needle slightly and inject the contents of the syringe.

Resistance vs Inference

- Slight resistance; congratulation, you have hit the right target
- Significant resistance; sorry, you have missed the target. Slightly withdraw, realign and inject

After care: At the injection site, after the injection:

- Apply icepacks
- Apply a firm sterile bandage under pressure.

Complications

- Infection (hence follow strict aseptic measures)
- Transient increase of pain (seen in 25% of the cases)
- Ecchymosis
- Haematoma formation.

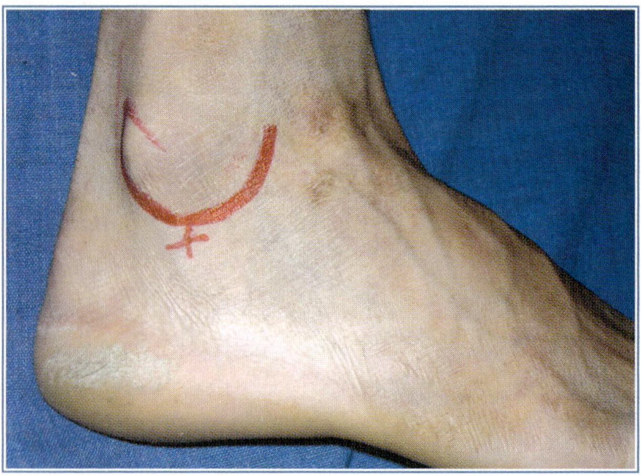

Fig. 4.31A: Insert the needle below the mid-point of the lateral malleolus

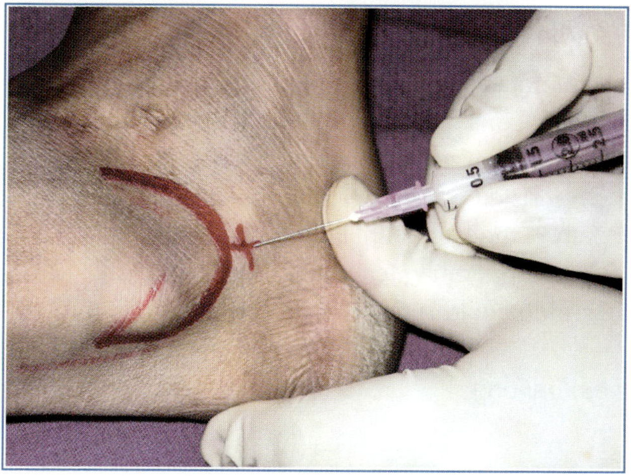

Fig. 4.31B: Insert the needle at a 30 degree angle to the lateral malleolus

Note: The incidence of ecchymosis and haematoma formation can be reduced if immediately after the injection, a firm sterile pressure bandage is applied.

Vital facts: Strictly observe the following after the injection:
- Simple analgesics and NSAIDs are advised
- To prevent the exacerbation of pain, avoid heat and gentle range of motion exercises for few days
- Avoid vigorous exercises for few days to prevent increase in pain.

Peroneal Tendinitis

Causes

- Repetitive trauma
- Everson injuries during running and playing tennis
- Improper stretching of the peroneal muscles prior to the exercise.

Presentation

- Acute onset of pain
- Pain is constant, severe and disturbs sleep
- Pain is localized to the posterior ankle
- On resisted eversion of the foot patient complains of pain in the lateral ankle and the foot
- Creaking, grating, crepitus could be heard
- Tendon could suddenly rupture.

Investigations

- Plain X-ray of the ankle
- Laboratory investigations
- MRI
- EMG
- Injection technique—both diagnostic and therapeutic
- Bone scan—to rule out stress fractures.

Preparation

- Position: Prone
- Drugs: 2 ml of 0.25 per cent preservative free bupivacaine and 40 mg of methylprednisolone
- Syringe: 5ml/1 ½ inches length and 25-gauge needle.

Techniques

- Put the patient in the above position
- Evert the foot strongly, identify the lower margin of the lateral malleolus

- Trace the path of the peroneal tendons anteriorly till the V-shaped division of the tendons is palpated
- Insert the needle at this point at a 30-degree angle to the ankle through the skin directed towards the lateral malleolus into the combined tendon sheath
- Inject the contents of the syringe gently into the tendon sheath.

Resistance vs Inference

- Slight resistance; congratulations you have hit the right target.
- Significant resistance; sorry, you have missed the target. Slightly withdraw, realign and inject.

Note: The successful injection is confirmed if the tendons distend into a dog-shaped appearance.

After care: At the injection site, after the injection:
- Apply icepacks
- Apply a firm sterile bandage under pressure.

Complications

- Infection (hence follow strict aseptic measures)
- Transient increase of pain (seen in 25% of the cases)
- Ecchymosis
- Haematoma formation.

Note: The incidence of ecchymosis and haematoma formation can be reduced if immediately after the injection, a firm sterile pressure bandage is applied.

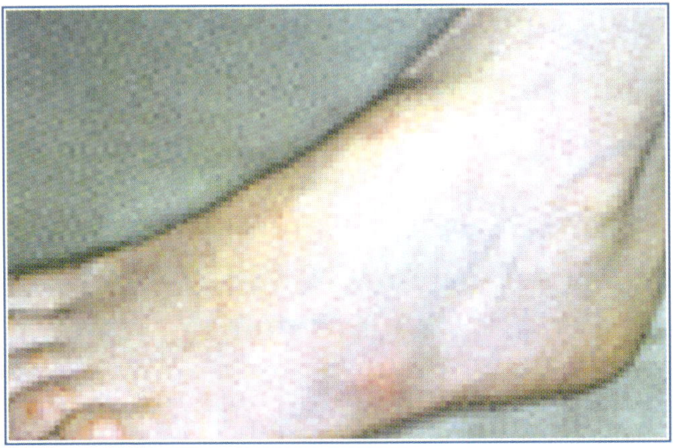

Fig. 4.32A: Clinical photograph of peroneal tendonitis

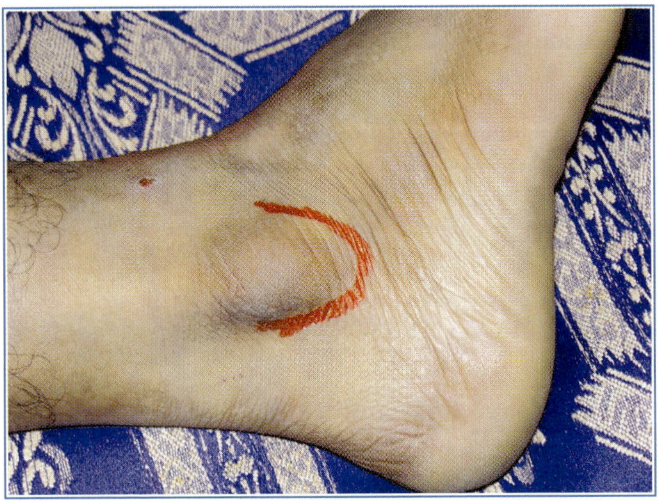

Fig. 4.32B: Identify and mark the lateral malleolus

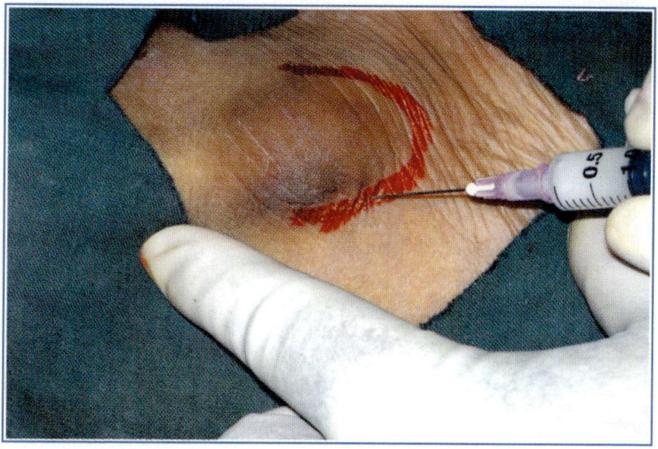

Fig. 4.32C: Insert the needle at 30 degrees to the ankle directed towards the lateral malleolus

Vital facts: Strictly observe the following after the injection:
- Simple analgesics and NSAIDs are advised
- To prevent the exacerbation of pain, avoid heat and gentle range of motion exercises for few days
- Avoid vigorous exercises for few days to prevent increase in pain.

Plantar Fascitis

It is an inflammation of the plantar fascia.

Causes

- Twice more common in women
- It can occur alone
- It can be part of rheumatoid arthritis, Reiter's syndrome or gout.

Predisposing Factors

- Obesity
- Bare foot walking
- Wearing house slippers for prolonged period
- High impact aerobic exercise.

Presentation

- Pain over the plantar surface of the calcaneum
- Pain is severe on first walking after nonweight bearing
- Pain becomes worse on prolonged standing or walking.

On Examination

- Point tenderness over the plantar medial calcaneal tuberosity
- Tenderness may be seen anteriorly along the plantar fascia
- Pain increases on dorsiflexion of the toes. This makes the plantar fascia taut and then palpating along the fascia from the heel to the forefoot.

Investigations

- Plain X-ray of the ankle
- Laboratory investigations
- MRI
- EMG
- Injection technique—both diagnostic and therapeutic
- Bone scan—to rule out stress fractures.

Preparation

- Position: Prone or lateral decubitus position with affected foot down.
- Drugs: 2 ml of 0.25 per cent preservative free bupivacaine and 40 mg of methylprednisolone
- Syringe: 2 ml/1 ½ inches length and 25-gauge needle.

Techniques

- Mark the two important landmarks
  a. Proximal base of the longitudinal arch at the medial side.
  b. Slightly distal to the medial process of the calcaneal tuberosity.
- Identify the most tender spot on the medial aspect of the heel by palpation. Mark this point
- Alternatively the site of pain can be approached directly from the plantar surface of the heel
- Advance the needle at 90 degrees to this point till it impinges on the bone
- Now withdraw the needle slowly and inject as close to the tender spot as possible.

Resistance vs Inference

- Slight resistance; congratulations you have hit the right target.
- Significant resistance; sorry, you have missed the target. Slightly withdraw, realign and inject.

After care: At the injection site, after the injection

- Apply icepacks
- Apply a firm sterile bandage under pressure.

Caution

- Do not inject into the fat pad
- Do not inject into the tibial nerve.

Complications

- Infection (hence follow strict aseptic measures)
- Rupture of plantar fascia
- Transient increase of pain (seen in 25% of the cases).

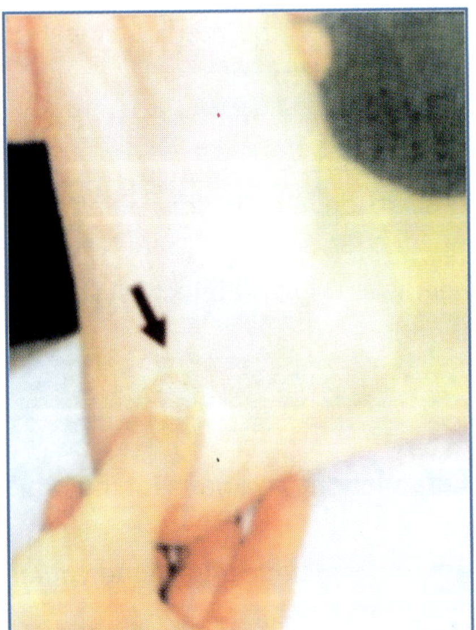

Fig. 4.33A: Method of eliciting tenderness in plantar fascia

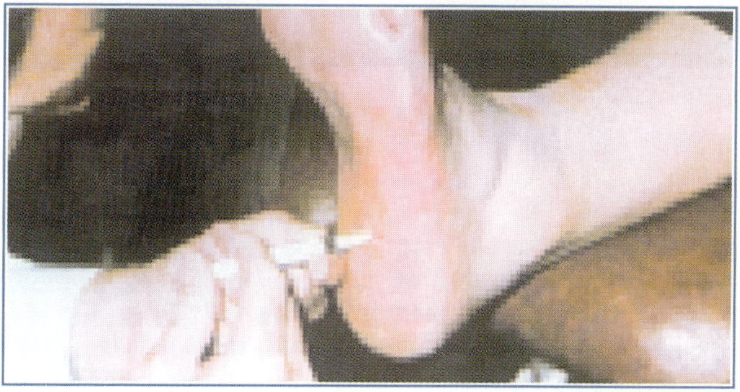

Fig. 4.33B: Method of giving injection through the plantar surface

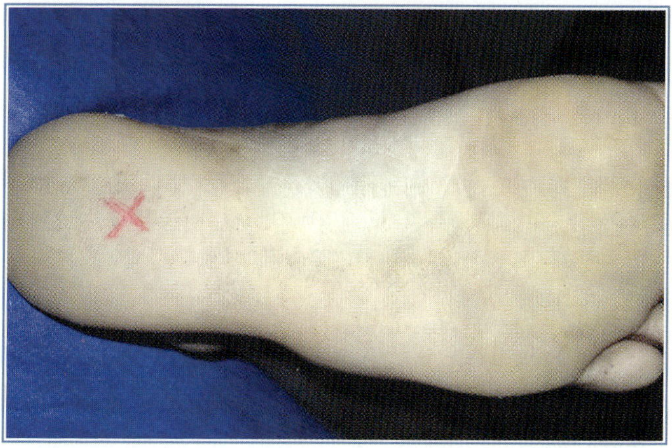

Fig. 4.33C: Mark the most tender spot over the plantar fascia

- Ecchymosis
- Haematoma formation
- Fat pad atrophy.

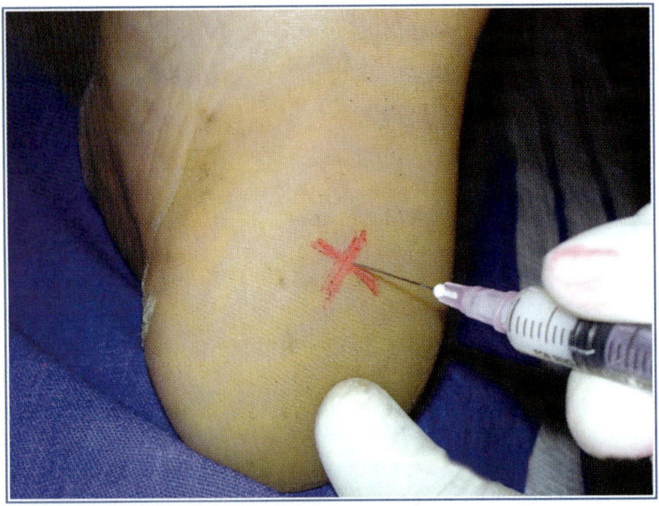

Fig. 4.33D: Insert the needle perpendicular to the skin through the marked spot

Note: The incidence of ecchymosis and haematoma formation can be reduced if immediately after the injection, a firm sterile pressure bandage is applied.

Vital facts: Strictly observe the following after the injection:

- Simple analgesics and NSAIDs are advised
- To prevent the exacerbation of pain, avoid heat and gentle range of motion exercises for few days
- Avoid vigorous exercises for few days to prevent increase in pain.

Calcaneal Spurs

These are usually associated with plantar fascitis.

Note: Though calcaneal spurs can occur anywhere along the calcaneum, it is most common at the insertion of the plantar fascia on the calcaneal tuberosity.

Causes

- Similar to plantar fascitis
- In some it could be due to excessive heel strike due to abnormal gait.

Presentation

Similar to plantar fascitis. In addition the pain of calcaneal spur is increased by weight bearing and by padding of the affected heel.

Investigations

- Plain X-ray of the ankle
- Laboratory investigations
- MRI
- EMG
- Injection technique—both diagnostic and therapeutic
- Bone scan—to rule out stress fractures.

Preparation

- Position: Prone
- Drugs: 2 ml of 0.25 per cent preservative free bupivacaine and 40 mg of methylprednisolone
- Syringe: 2 ml/1 ½ inches length and 25-gauge needle.

Techniques

- Identify the painful area of the heel by careful palpation
- Insert the needle at 90 degrees to this point, directed towards the center of the painful area until it impinges the bone
- With draw and re-inject.

Resistance vs Inference

- Slight resistance; congratulations you have hit the right target.
- Significant resistance; sorry, you have missed the target. Slightly withdraw, realign and inject.

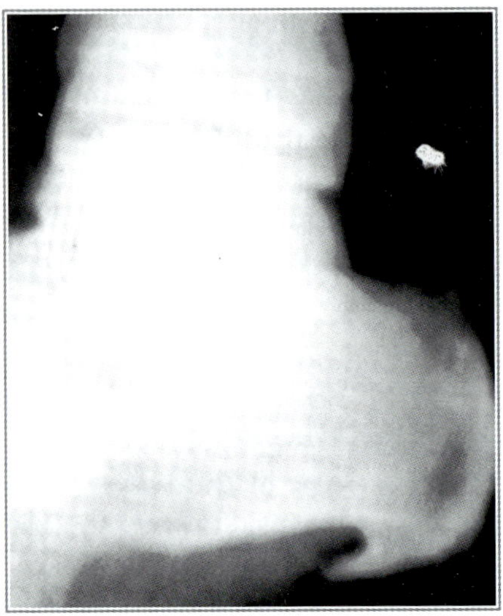

Fig. 4.34A: Plain X-ray of the heel showing prominent calcaneal spur

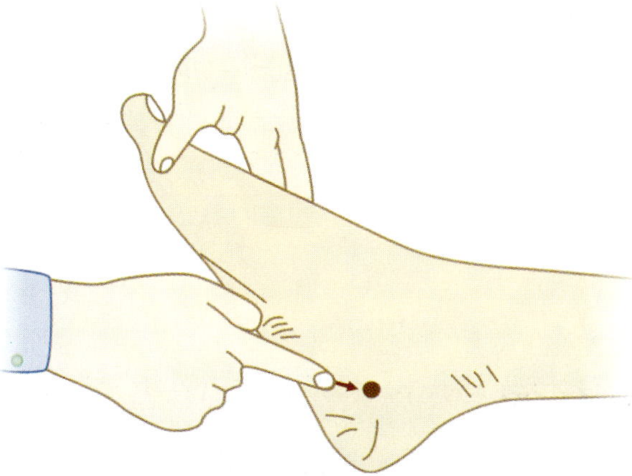

Fig. 4.34B: Point of tenderness in calcaneal spur

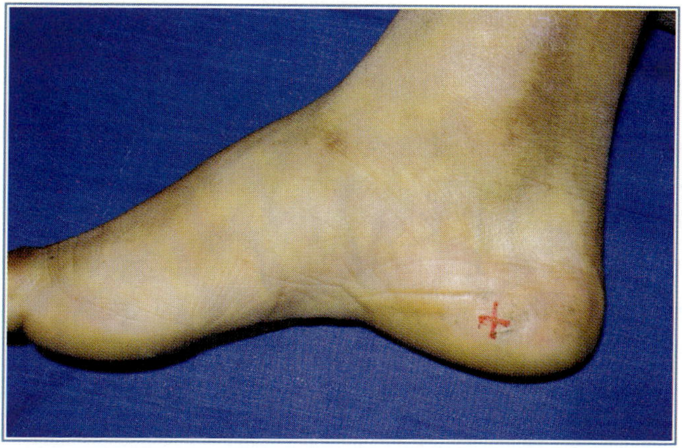

Fig. 4.34C: Mark the tender spot on the medial side of the heel

After care: At the injection site, after the injection:

- Apply icepacks
- Apply a firm sterile bandage under pressure.

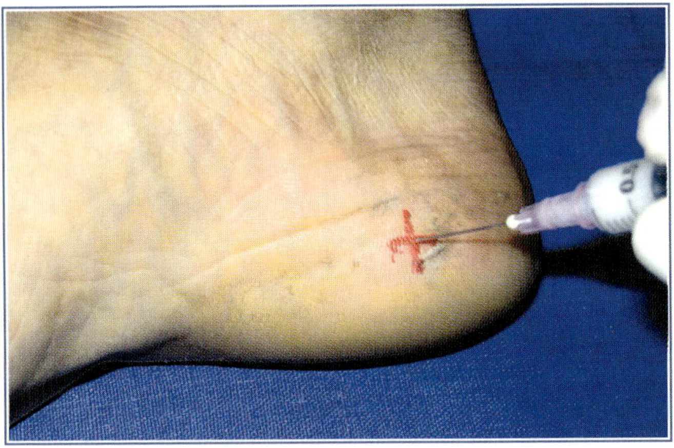

Fig. 4.34D: Insert the needle perpendicular to the skin towards the tender spot

Complications

- Infection (hence follow strict aseptic measures)
- Transient increase of pain (seen in 25% of the cases)
- Ecchymosis
- Haematoma formation.

Note: The incidence of ecchymosis and haematoma formation can be reduced if immediately after the injection, a firm sterile pressure bandage is applied.

Vital facts: Strictly observe the following after the injection:
- Simple analgesics and NSAIDs are advised
- To prevent the exacerbation of pain, avoid heat and gentle range of motion exercises for few days
- Avoid vigorous exercises for few days to prevent increase in pain.

Retrocalcaneal Spur

This is a bony outgrowth developing from the posterior tuberosity of the calcaneum. Less common than the calcaneal spur and injection treatment gives considerable relief in these cases.

Retrocalcaneal Bursitis

Due to repeated friction with the edges of a pump shows adventitious bursa may develop over the posterior aspect of the heel also called as 'pump-bump' and injection treatment helps.

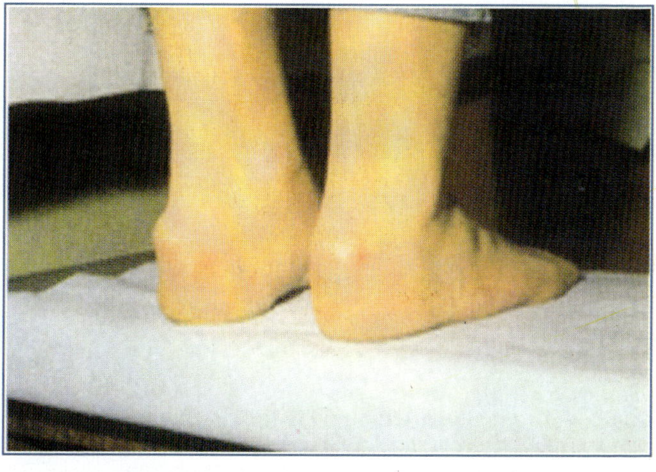

Fig. 4.35A: Clinical photograph of retrocalcaneal spur

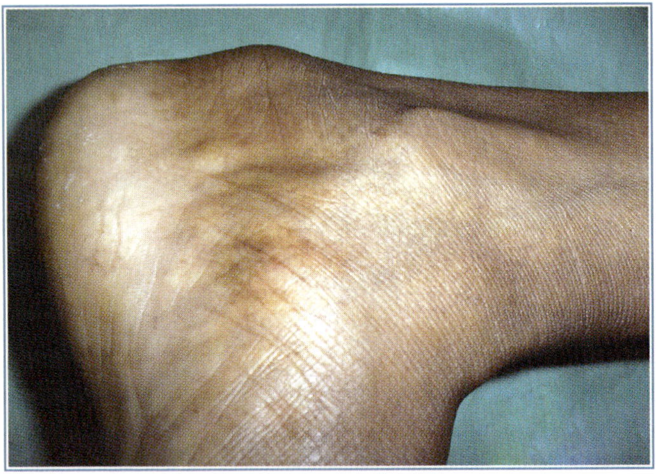

Fig. 4.35B: Showing a prominent RC spur

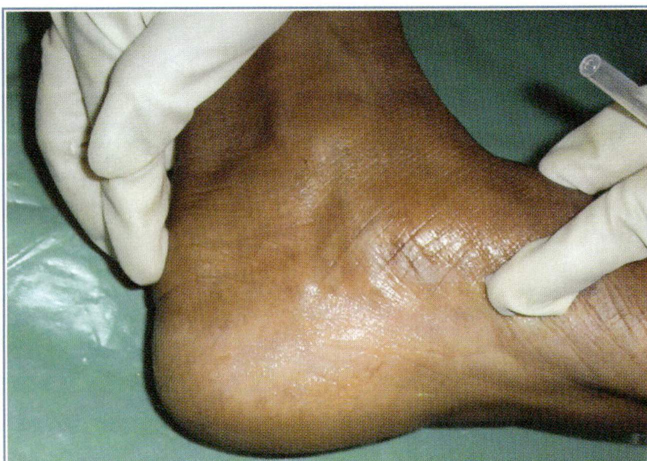

Fig. 4.35C: Palpate the spur and mark it

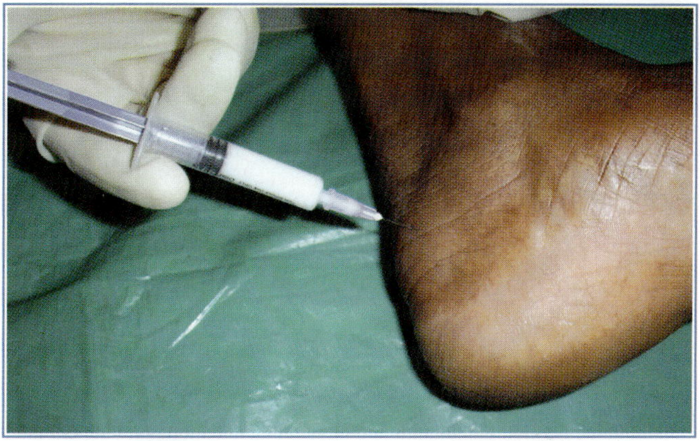

Fig. 4.35D: Inject over the most tender spot over the spur

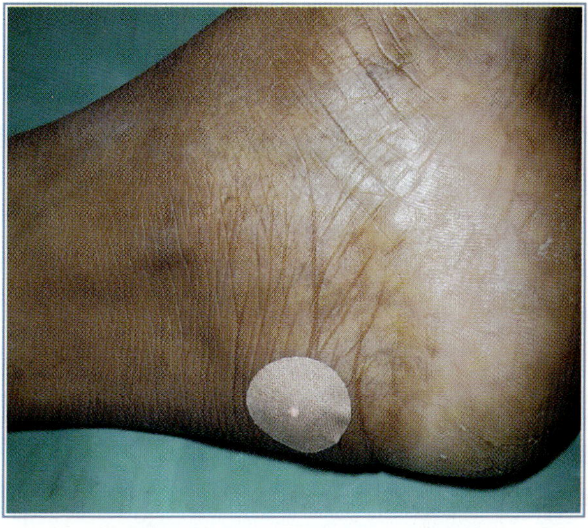

Fig. 4.35E: Seal the injection point with a sterile bandaid

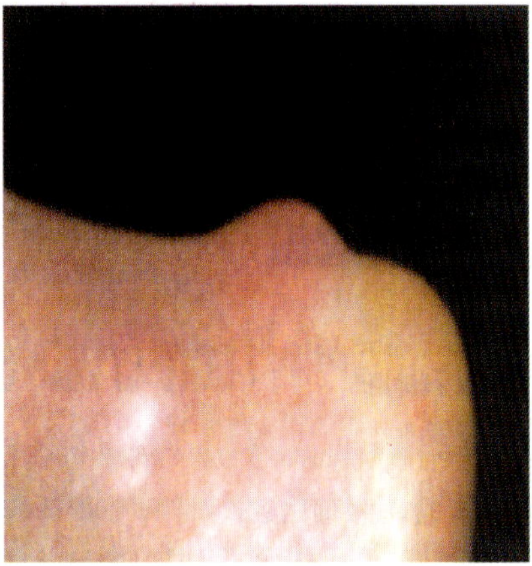

Fig. 4.36A: Clinical photograph of Retrocalcaneal bursitis

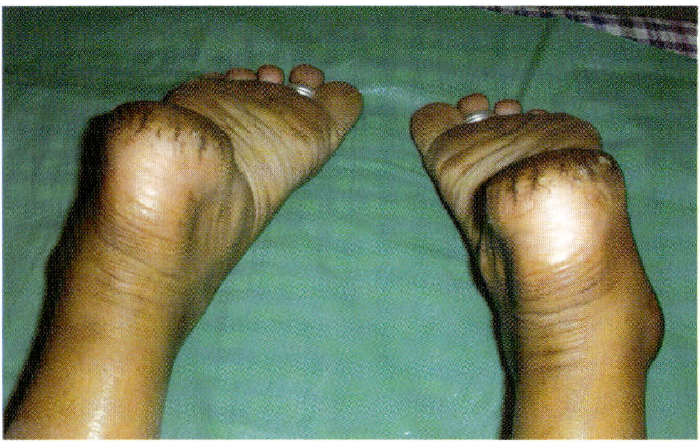

Fig. 4.36B: Showing bilateral retrocalcaneal bursitis

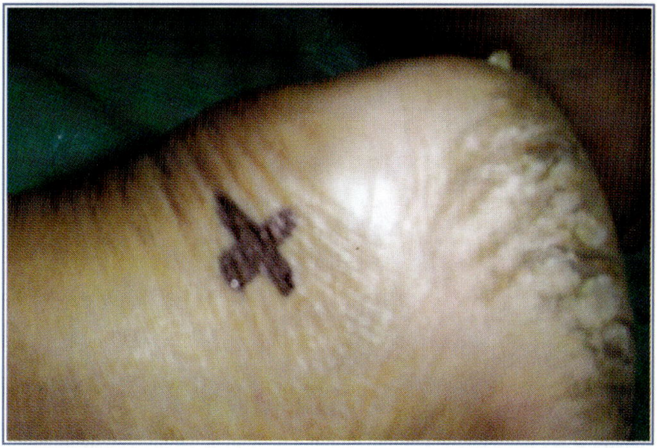

Fig. 4.36C: Mark the tender spot with a sterile marker

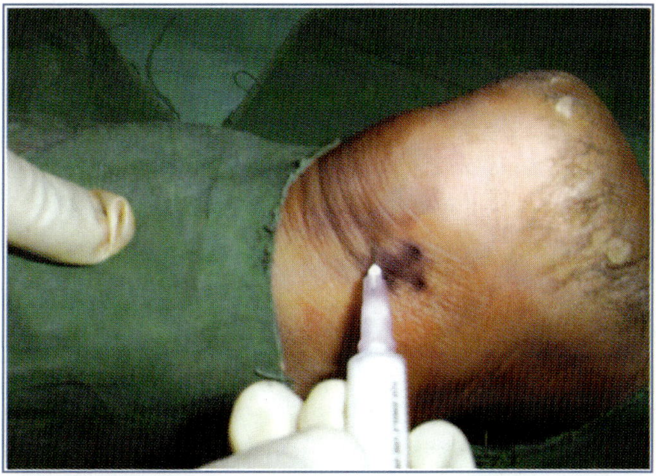

Fig. 4.36D: Advance the needle perpendicular to the Achilles tendon into the bursa

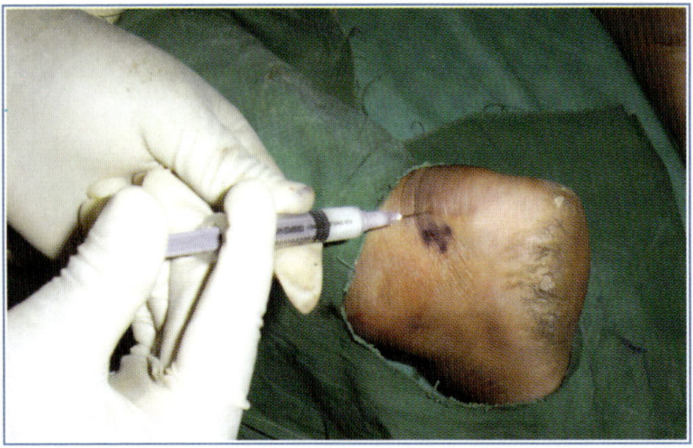

Fig. 4.36E: Alternatively the needle can be inserted through the center of the bursa

Posterior Tibialis Tendinitis

Causes

- Acute eversion injury
- Fractures of the ankle.

Presentation

- Pain is constant and severe and is localized to the inner aspect of the ankle
- Patient complains that the inside of the ankles is rubbing with their shoes raw and on examination the skin appears normal
- Pain interferes with sleep

- Antalgic gait is seen
- Pain increases on resisted inversion and passive eversion of the ankle
- The ankle may feel hot and appear swollen
- While passively inverting or everting the ankle there could be a creaking or grating sensation.

Investigations

- Plain X-ray of the ankle
- Laboratory investigations
- MRI
- EMG
- Injection technique—both diagnostic and therapeutic
- Bone scan—to rule out stress fractures.

Preparation

- Position: Supine
- Drugs: 2 ml of 0.25 per cent preservative free bupivacaine and 40 mg of methylprednisolone
- Syringe: 5 ml/1 ½ inches length and 25-gauge needle.

Techniques

- Patient is in the above position
- The lower limb is slightly abducted
- Identify the lower margin of the medial malleolus. Mark this point.
- Insert the needle at this point at an angle of 30 degrees to the ankle till it impinges against the lower margin of the medial malleolus

- Withdraw the needle and inject the contents of the syringe slowly.

Resistance vs Inference

- Slight resistance; congratulations you have hit the right target
- Significant resistance; sorry, you have missed the target. Slightly withdraw, realign and inject.

After care: At the injection site, after the injection
- Apply icepacks
- Apply a firm sterile bandage under pressure.

Complications

- Infection (hence follow strict aseptic measures)
- Transient increase of pain (seen in 25% of the cases)
- Ecchymosis
- Haematoma formation.

Note: The incidence of ecchymosis and haematoma formation can be reduced if immediately after the injection, a firm sterile pressure bandage is applied.

Vital facts: Strictly observe the following after the injection:
- Simple analgesics and NSAIDs are advised
- To prevent the exacerbation of pain, avoid heat and gentle range of motion exercises for few days
- Avoid vigorous exercises for few days to prevent increase in pain.

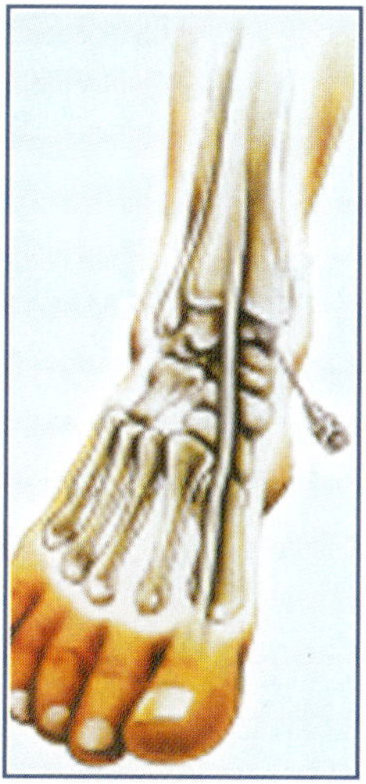

Fig. 4.37A: Approach towards the medial side of the ankle

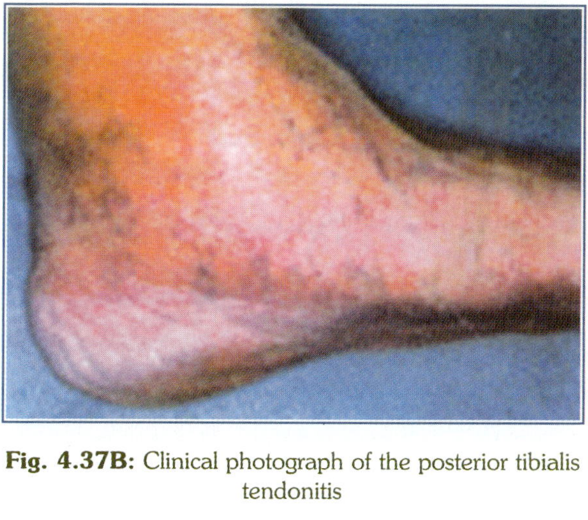

Fig. 4.37B: Clinical photograph of the posterior tibialis tendonitis

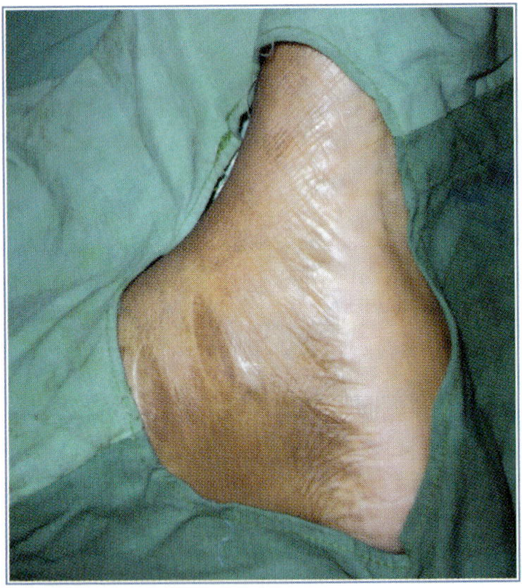

Fig. 4.37C: Paint and drape the area

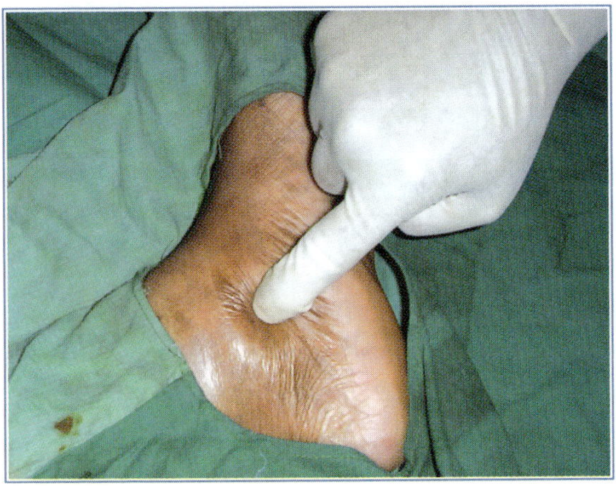

Fig. 4.37D: Palpate the most tender spot just below the medial malleolus

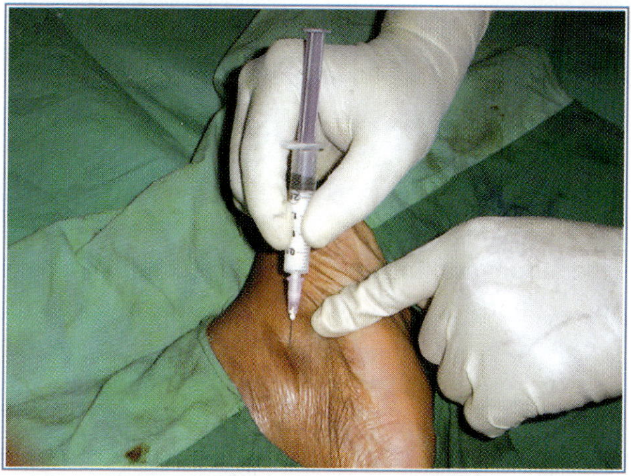

Fig. 4.37E: Insert the needle in a 30-degree direction towards the medial malleolus

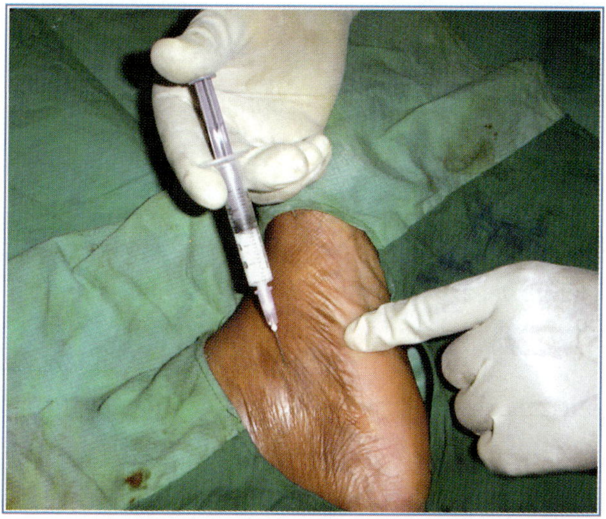

Fig. 4.37F: Inject the contents of the syringe

BUNION PAIN SYNDROME

Bunion involves the following:

- Soft tissue swelling of the first metatarsophalangeal joint
- Abnormal angulations of the first metatarsophalangeal joint
- Prominent first metatarsal head
- Overlapping of the first and second toes
- Adventitious bursa may develop over the bunion.

Causes

- More common in women
- Seen in people who wear tight fitting narrow toed shoes
- High heeled shoes may increase the problem.

Presentation

- Pain over the first metatarsophalangeal joint
- Difficulty in wearing the shoes
- Walking increases the pain
- Pain is constant and dull aching and interferes with sleep
- There could be crepitus, grating or popping sensation
- Hallux valgus deformity develops over the years
- Rest and heel decreases the pain.

Investigations

- Plain X-ray of the ankle
- Laboratory investigations
- MRI

- EMG
- Injection technique—both diagnostic and therapeutic
- Bone scan—to rule out stress fractures.

Preparation

- Position: Supine
- Drugs: 2 ml of 0.25 per cent preservative free bupivacaine and 40 mg of methylprednisolone
- Syringe: 2 ml/5/8 inches length and 25-gauge needle.

Techniques

- Paint and drape the area
- Identify the bunion
- Insert the needle against the first metatarsal head till it hits the bone
- Withdraw the needle slightly and inject the contents of the syringe.

Resistance vs Inference

- Slight resistance; congratulations you have hit the right target.
- Significant resistance; sorry, you have missed the target. Slightly withdraw, realign and inject.

After care: At the injection site, after the injection:

- Apply icepacks
- Apply a firm sterile bandage under pressure.

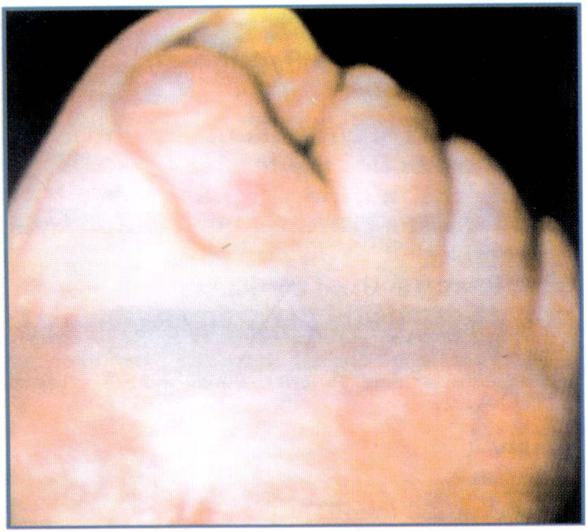

Fig. 4.38A: Clinical photograph of hallux valgus and bunion

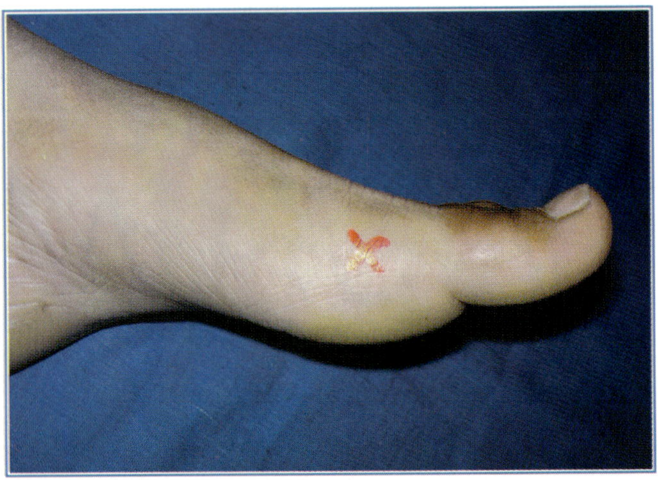

Fig. 4.38B: Identify and mark the most prominent part on the medial side of the first metarsophalangeal joint

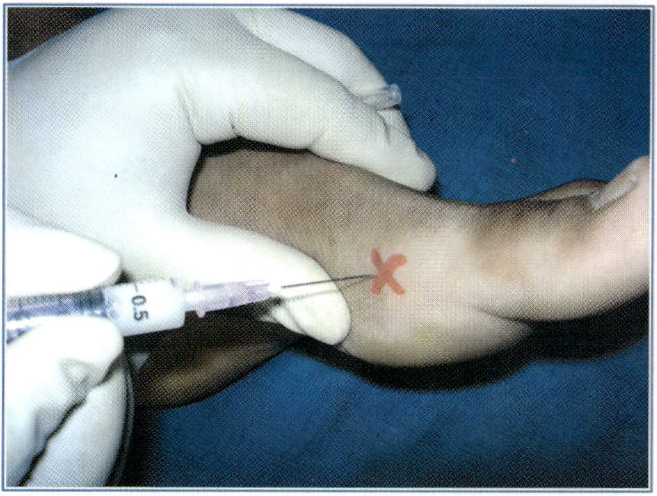

Fig. 4.38C: Insert the needle at right angles at the point marked above

Complications

- Infection (hence follow strict aseptic measures)
- Transient increase of pain (seen in 25% of the cases)
- Ecchymosis
- Haematoma formation.

Note: The incidence of ecchymosis and haematoma formation can be reduced if immediately after the injection, a firm sterile pressure bandage is applied.

Vital facts: Strictly observe the following after the injection:
- Simple analgesics and NSAIDs are advised
- To prevent the exacerbation of pain, avoid heat and gentle range of motion exercises for few days
- Avoid vigorous exercises for few days to prevent increase in pain.

Bunionette Pain Syndrome (Tailor's Bunion)

Bunionette involves the following:

- Soft tissue swelling over the 5th metatarsophalangeal joint
- Abnormal angulation of the joint
- Prominent 5th metatarsal head
- Medial angulation of the little toe
- A corn could also develop.

Causes

- Common in females
- Most common cause is wearing of tight narrow shoes
- High heeled shoes increases the problem.

Presentation

- Pain over the fifth metatarsophalangeal joint
- Difficulty to wear the shoes
- Walking increases the pain
- Rest and heat decreases the pain
- Pain may interfere with sleep
- Grating, popping or crepitus sensation could be heard
- Medial angulation deformity of the little toe may develop.

Investigations

- Plain X-ray of the ankle
- Laboratory investigations

- MRI
- EMG
- Injection technique—both diagnostic and therapeutic
- Bone scan—to rule out stress fractures.

Preparation

- Position: Supine
- Drugs: 2 ml of 0.25 per cent preservative free bupivacaine and 40 mg of methylprednisolone
- Syringe: 2 ml/5/8 inches length and 25-gauge needle.

Techniques

- Paint and drape the area
- Identify the bunion
- Insert the needle against the fifth metatarsal head till it hits the bone
- Withdraw the needle slightly and inject the contents of the syringe.

Resistance vs Inference

- Slight resistance; congratulation, you have hit the right target
- Significant resistance; sorry, you have missed the target. Slightly withdraw, realign and inject.

After care: At the injection site, after the injection:

- Apply icepacks
- Apply a firm sterile bandage under pressure.

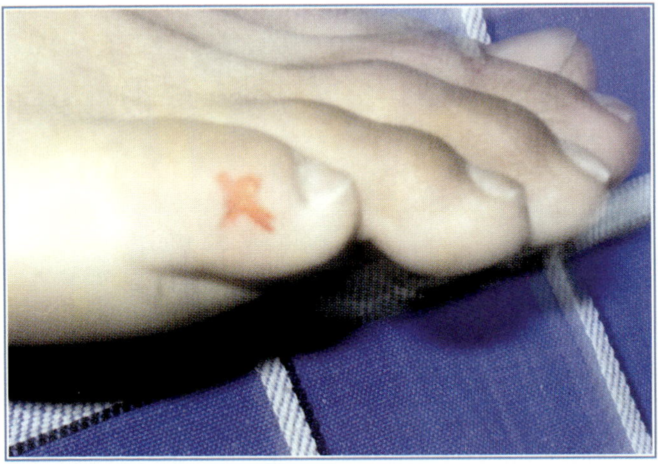

Fig. 4.39A: Identify the fifth metatarsal head and mark the most tender point over the bunionette

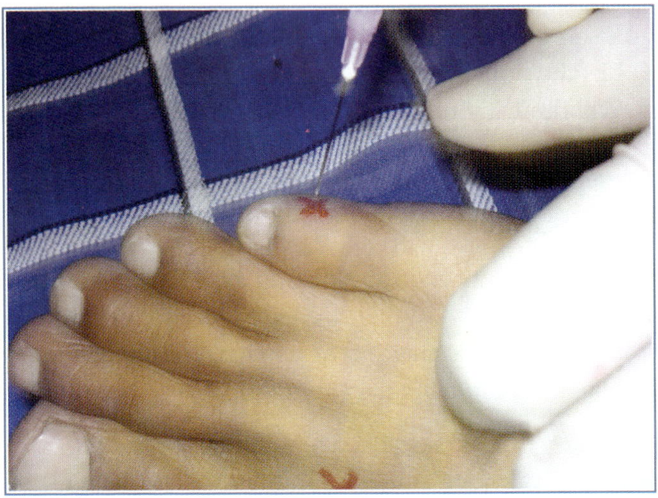

Fig. 4.39B: Insert the needle at right angle to the marked point above

Complications

- Infection (hence follow strict aseptic measures)
- Transient increase of pain (seen in 25% of the cases)
- Ecchymosis
- Haematoma formation.

Note: The incidence of ecchymosis and haematoma formation can be reduced if immediately after the injection, a firm sterile pressure bandage is applied.

Vital facts: Strictly observe the following after the injection:
- Simple analgesics and NSAIDs are advised
- To prevent the exacerbation of pain, avoid heat and gentle range of motion exercises for few days
- Avoid vigorous exercises for few days to prevent increase in pain.

Mallet Toe Pain Syndrome

This consists of:
- Painful flexion deformity of the DIP joint
- Second toe is most commonly affected
- It is most common in females
- A painful adventitious bursa may develop
- A callus or ulcer may develop over the tip of the affected toe.

Causes

- Jamming injury to the second toe
- Ill fitting, tight, narrow shoes
- High heeled shoes may exacerbate the problem.

Presentation

- Pain is localized to the affected toe
- Walking increases the pain, rest and heat relieves the pain
- Pain is constant and dull aching
- Patient complains of inability to wear and fit the shoes
- Crepitus, grating or popping sensation could be heard
- Characteristic flexion deformity may develop in the later stages.

Note: Unlike in bunion, alignment of the toes is not affected.

Investigations

- Plain X-ray of the ankle
- Laboratory investigations
- MRI
- EMG
- Injection technique—both diagnostic and therapeutic
- Bone scan—to rule out stress fractures.

Preparation

- Position: Supine
- Drugs: 2 ml of 0.25 per cent preservative free bupivacaine and 40 mg of methylprednisolone
- Syringe: 2 ml/5/8 inches length and 25-gauge needle.

Techniques

- Identify the mallet toe
- The needle is inserted into the affected distal phalanges till it hits the bone

- Now slightly withdraw the needle and inject the contents of the syringe.

Resistance vs Inference

- Slight resistance; congratulations you have hit the right target.
- Significant resistance; sorry, you have missed the target. Slightly withdraw, realign and inject.

After care: At the injection site, after the injection:

- Apply icepacks
- Apply a firm sterile bandage under pressure.

Complications

- Infection (hence follow strict aseptic measures)
- Transient increase of pain (seen in 25% of the cases)
- Ecchymosis
- Haematoma formation.

Note: The incidence of ecchymosis and haematoma formation can be reduced if immediately after the injection, a firm sterile pressure bandage is applied.

Vital facts: Strictly observe the following after the injection:

- Simple analgesics and NSAIDs are advised
- To prevent the exacerbation of pain, avoid heat and gentle range of motion exercises for few days
- Avoid vigorous exercises for few days to prevent increase in pain.

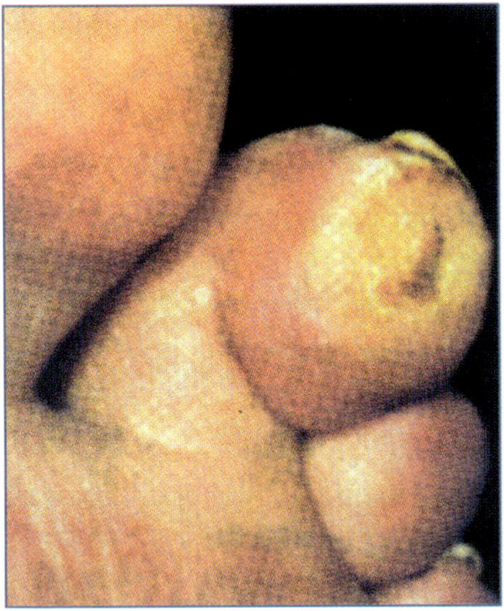

Fig. 4.40A: Clinical photograph showing mallet toe

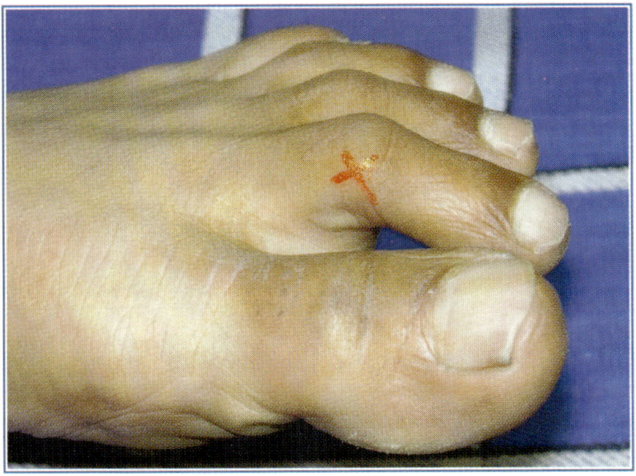

Fig. 4.40B: Mark the affected phalanx

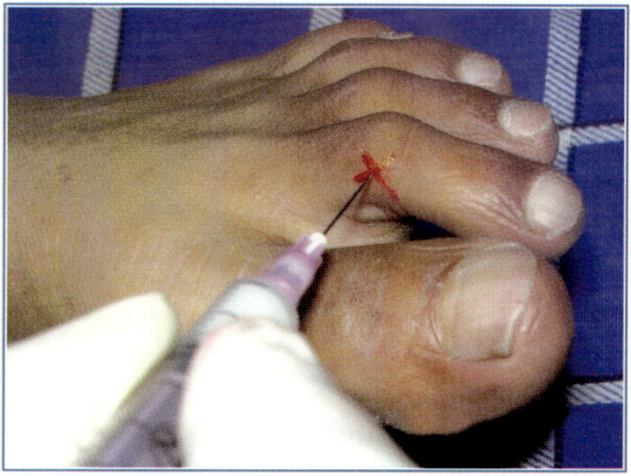

Fig. 4.40C: Inject into the affected phalanx

Hammer Toe Pain Syndrome

This Syndrome consists of:

- Painful flexion deformity of the PIP joint
- Second toe is affected the most
- It is usually bilateral
- It is more common in females.

Causes

- It is due to wearing too tight shoes
- Trauma to the foot
- High heels increases the pain.

Presentation

- Pain that is localized to the affected PIP joint
- Walking increases the pain, rest and heat relieves it

- Pain may interfere with sleep
- Grating, crepitus or popping sensation could be heard
- Typical hammer toe pain develops in the late stages
- Inability to wear the shoes.

Investigations

- Plain X-ray of the ankle
- Laboratory investigations
- MRI
- EMG
- Injection technique—both diagnostic and therapeutic
- Bone scan—to rule out stress fractures.

Preparation

- Position: Supine
- Drugs: 2 ml of 0.25 per cent preservative free bupivacaine and 40 mg of methylprednisolone
- Syringe: 2 ml/5/8 inches length and 25-gauge needle.

Procedures

- Identify the hammer toe
- The needle is advanced slowly into the skin against the second metatarsal head
- Withdraw the needle and inject.

After care: At the injection site, after the injection:

- Apply icepacks
- Apply a firm sterile bandage under pressure.

Complications

- Infection (hence follow strict aseptic measures)
- Transient increase of pain (seen in 25% of the cases)
- Ecchymosis
- Haematoma formation.

Note: The incidence of ecchymosis and haematoma formation can be reduced if immediately after the injection, a firm sterile pressure bandage is applied.

Vital facts: Strictly observe the following after the injection:
- Simple analgesics and NSAIDs are advised
- To prevent the exacerbation of pain, avoid heat and gentle range of motion exercises for few days
- Avoid vigorous exercises for few days to prevent increase in pain.

Resistance vs Inference

- Slight resistance; congratulations you have hit the right target.
- Significant resistance; sorry, you have missed the target. Slightly withdraw, realign and inject.

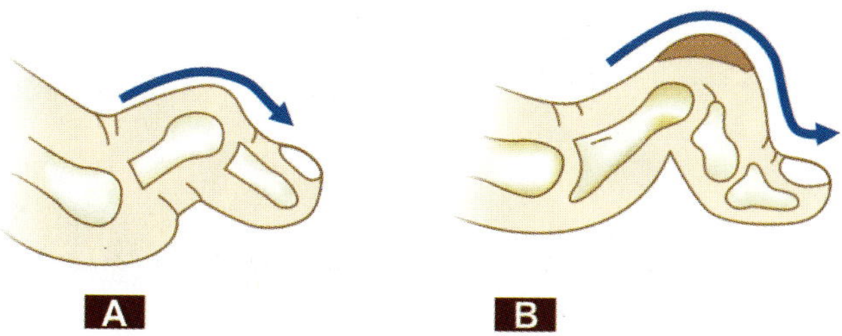

Fig. 4.41A: Showing hammer toe (A) and claw toes (B)

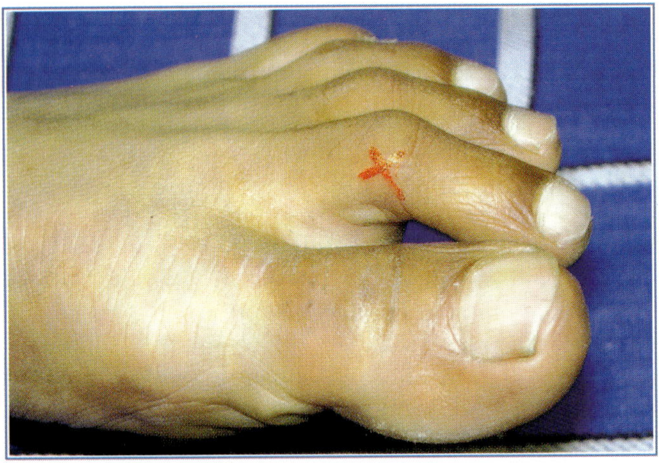

Fig. 4.41B: Identify the mallet/hammer toe

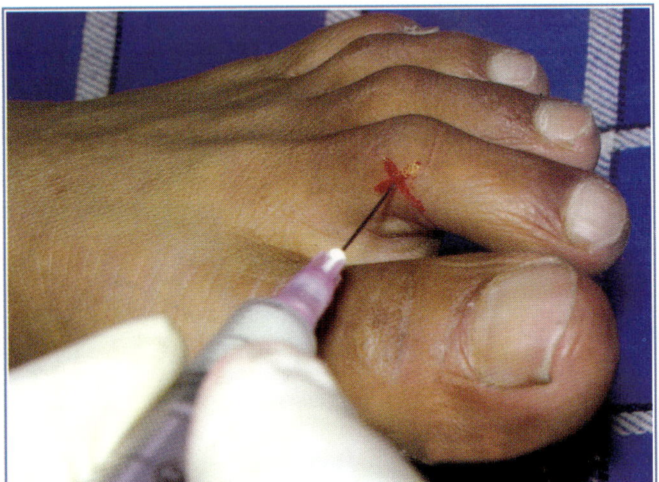

Fig. 4.41C: The needle is inserted into the deformed toe at right angle and injected

Morton's Neuroma Pain

This is characterized by:

- It is the most common pain syndrome that affects the forefoot
- It is believed to be due to perineural fibrosis of the interdigital nerve
- The nerve between the 3rd and 4th toes are most commonly affected
- It is usually due to wearing of right and arrow shoes.

Presentation

- Patient complains of burning pain in the plantar surface of the foot
- Painful paraesthesiae into the affected two toes
- Patient feels a sensation of walking with a stone in the shoes
- Pain increases with prolonged standing or walking
- Pain increases with wearing improperly fitting shoes.

Signs

- Antalgic gait
- Forefoot compression test: Compress the forefoot with one hand firmly while the other hand firmly presses on the interdigital space. Pain with paraesthesiae radiating into the two affected toes is reproduced.

Note: In metatarsalgia, pain may remains on the metatarsal heads.

Investigations

- Plain X-ray of the ankle
- Laboratory investigations
- MRI
- EMG
- Injection technique—both diagnostic and therapeutic
- Bone scan—to rule out stress fractures.

Preparation

- Position: Supine position with foot in neutral position and knees slightly flexed over a towel roll
- Drugs: 3 ml of norepinephrine containing lignocaine and 40 mg of methylprednisolone
- Syringe: 12 ml/ 1 and ½ inches length and 25- to 27-gauze needle.

Techniques

- Patient is put in the above position
- The area is painted and draped
- The affected interdigital space is identified and the dorsal surface of the foot at the point of maximum tenderness is marked with a sterile marker
- Insert the needle at this point proximal to the metatarsal head, insert the needle inbetween the metatarsal bones
- Advance the needle 45° proximally directed towards the heel from the dorsal to palmar surface while slowly injecting the drug.

Resistance and Inference

- Slight resistance; congratulation you have hit the right target.
- Significant resistance; sorry, you have missed the target. Slightly withdraw, realign and inject.

After care: At the injection site, after the injection:
- Apply icepacks
- Apply a firm sterile bandage under pressure.

Caution

Do not inject into plantar fat pad.

Complications

- Infection (hence follow strict aseptic measures)
- Transient increase of pain (seen in 25% of the cases)
- Ecchymosis
- Haematoma formation
- Plantar fat pad atrophy.

Note: The incidence of ecchymosis and haematoma formation can be reduced if immediately after the injection, a firm sterile pressure bandage is applied.

Vital facts: Strictly observe the following after the injection:
- Simple analgesics and NSAIDs are advised
- To prevent the exacerbation of pain, avoid heat and gentle range of motion exercises for few days
- Avoid vigorous exercises for few days to prevent increase in pain.

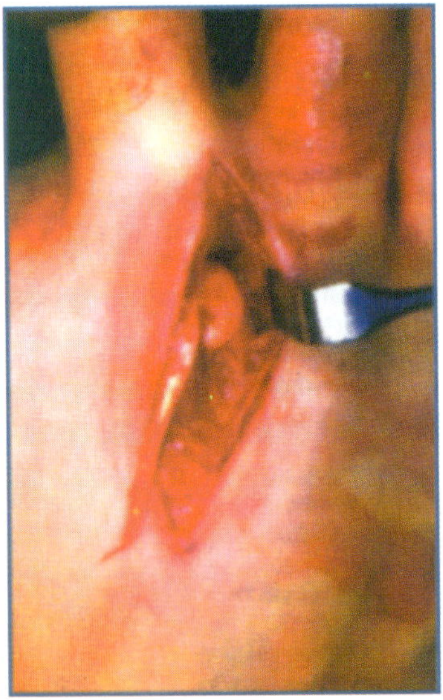

Fig. 4.42A: Clinical photograph of Morton neuroma

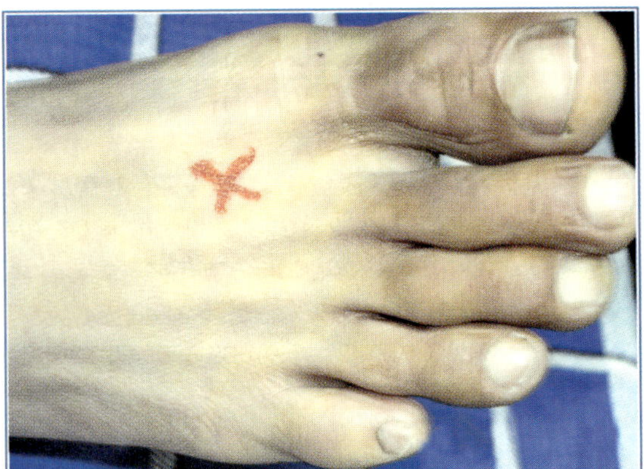

Fig. 4.42B: Identify the most tender point in the interdigital space and mark it

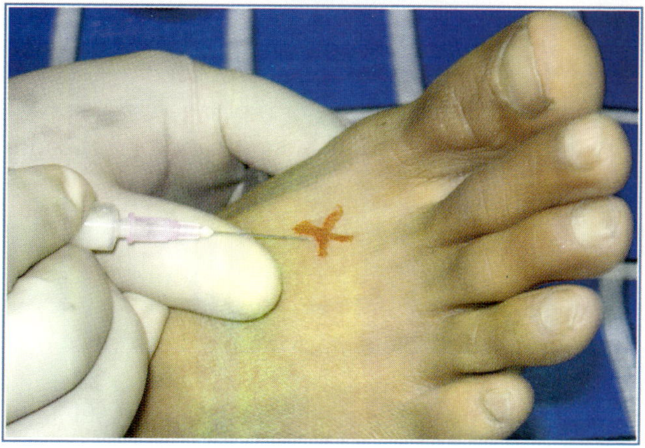

Fig. 4.42C: Insert the needle at this point

Sesamoiditis

Features

- It is charactised by pain and tenderness over the metatarsal head
- First sesamoid bone over the first metatarsal bone is affected the most, followed by the second and fifth metatarsal heads
- There is a sensation of walking with a stone in the shoes.

Causes

- It is due to pushing off injuries during foot ball
- Due to repetitive microtrauma from running or dancing.

Features

- Pain is felt over the first metatarsal head
- Pain increases on walking or prolonged standing
- It increases by wearing ill fitting or improperly padded shoes.

Signs

- Antalgic gait is present
- Ecchymosis is present over the plantar surface of the foot
- Tenderness over the sesamoid bone. Here the tender area moves with the flexor tendons when the patient actively flexes the toes.

Note: In metatarsalgia pain tenderness remains over the metatarsal heads.

Investigations

- Plain X-ray of the ankle
- Laboratory investigations
- MRI
- EMG
- Injection technique—both diagnostic and therapeutic
- Bone scan—to rule out stress fractures.

Preparation

- Position: Supine position
- Drugs: 2 ml of preservative free bupivacaine and 40 mg of methylprednisolone
- Syringe: 2 ml, 5/8 inches length and 25-gauge needle.

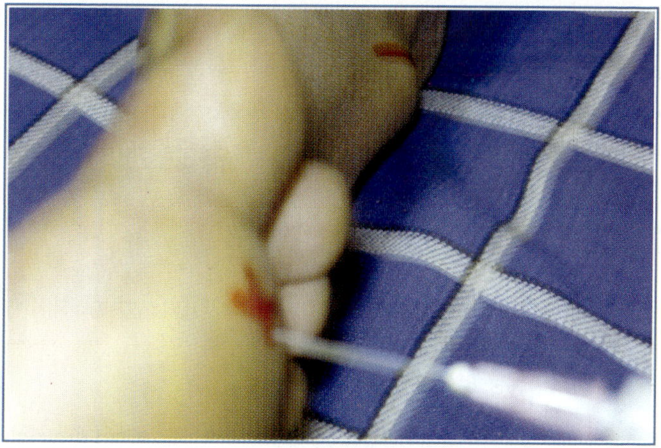

Fig. 4.43A: Identify and mark the affected sesamoid bone

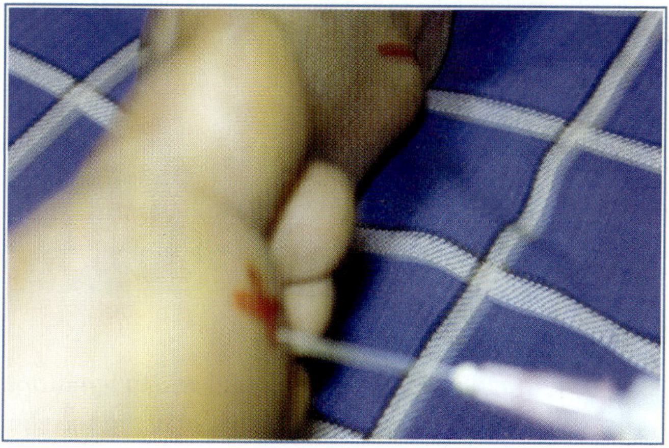

Fig. 4.43B: Insert the needle at this point

Techniques

- Patient is put in the above position
- Identify the affected sesamoid bone
- Insert the needle towards the affected sesamoid bone through the plantar surface
- Now slightly withdraw the needle
- Do a test aspirate for blood
- If test is negative inject the contents of the syringe slowly.

Resistance vs Inference

- Slight resistance; congratulations you have hit the right target.
- Significant resistance; sorry, you have missed the target. Slightly withdraw, realign and inject.

After care: At the injection site, after the injection

- Apply icepacks
- Apply a firm sterile bandage under pressure.

Complications

- Infection (hence follow strict aseptic measures)
- Transient increase of pain (seen in 25% of the cases)
- Ecchymosis
- Haematoma formation.

Note: The incidence of ecchymosis and haematoma formation can be reduced if immediately after the injection, a firm sterile pressure bandage is applied.

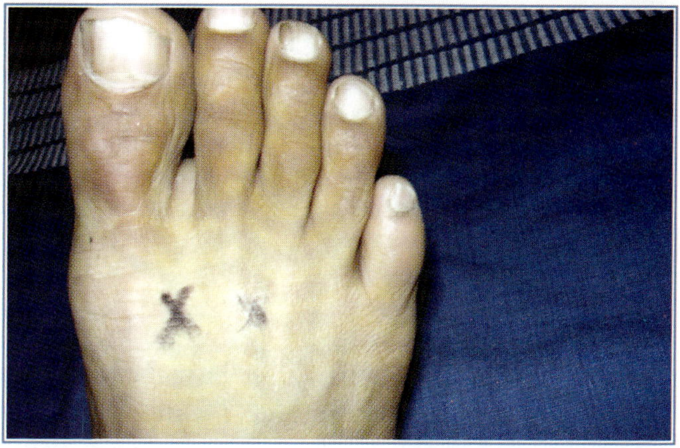

Fig. 4.44A: Identify the affected metatarsal head. Mark the most tender spot with a sterile marker

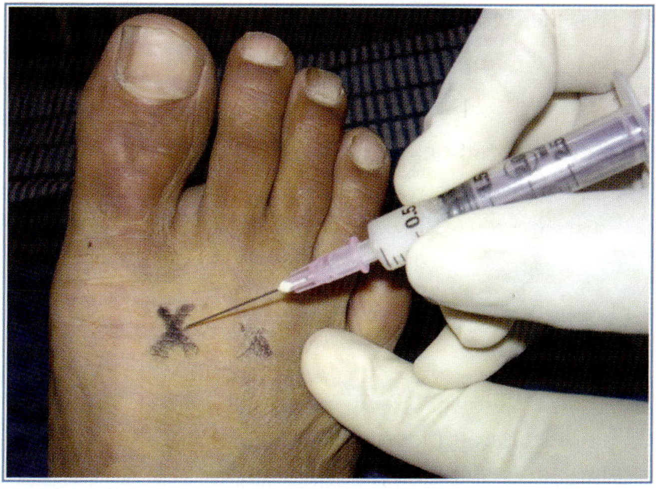

Fig. 4.44B: Insert the needle over the dorsal surface of the foot next to the affected metatarsal head

Vital facts: Strictly observe the following after the injection:
- Simple analgesics and NSAIDs are advised
- To prevent the exacerbation of pain, avoid heat and gentle range of motion exercises for few days
- Avoid vigorous exercises for few days to prevent increase in pain.

Metatarsalgia

Features

- Tenderness and pain present over the metatarsal heads
- Feeling of walking with a stone in the shoes
- Hence callus could develop over the heads of the second and third metatarsals due to shifting off weight from the first metatarsal head to relieve pain
- This callus further exacerbates the pain due to pressure.

Presentation

- Pain over the metatarsal head
- Pain increases on walking for long distances
- Pain increases by wearing tight fitting improper footwear.

Signs

- Antalgic gain is present
- Tenderness on pressing the metatarsal heads
- Flattening of the arch could develop
- Callus formation is seen.

Note: The callus is differentiated from the wart by the absence of thrombosed blood vessels that appear as small, dark spots through the substance of the wart when the surface is trimmed.

Investigations

- Plain X-ray of the ankle
- Laboratory investigations
- MRI
- EMG
- Injection technique—both diagnostic and therapeutic
- Bone scan—to rule out stress fractures.

Preparation

- Position: Supine position
- Drugs: 2 ml of preservative free bupivacaine and 40 mg of methylprednisolone
- Syringe: 2 ml, 5/8 inches length and 25-gauge needle.

Techniques

- Paint and drape the area
- Identify the affected metatarsal head. Mark the point with a sterile marker
- Insert the needle over the dorsal surface of the foot to a depth of ½ inches from the skin
- If you hit the bone, withdraw and redirect it more laterally

- Place the needle next to the affected metatarsal head and do an aspiration test for the blood
- If the above test is negative, inject the contents of the syringe gently.

Resistance and Inference

- Slight resistance; congratulation, you have hit the right target.
- Significant resistance; sorry, you have missed the target. Slightly withdraw, realign and inject.

After care: At the injection site, after the injection

- Apply icepacks
- Apply a firm sterile bandage under pressure.

Complications

- Infection (hence follow strict aseptic measures)
- Transient increase of pain (seen in 25% of the cases)
- Ecchymosis
- Haematoma formation.

Note: The incidence of ecchymosis and haematoma formation can be reduced if immediately after the injection, a firm sterile pressure bandage is applied.

Vital facts: Strictly observe the following after the injection:

- Simple analgesics and NSAIDs are advised
- To prevent the exacerbation of pain, avoid heat and gentle range of motion exercises for few days
- Avoid vigorous exercises for few days to prevent increase in pain.

Index

H

I

J

K

L

M

O

P

Q

R

S

T

U

X